<u>HERBAL MEDICINE</u>

Herbal Antibiotics ,The Ultimate Guide Guide to Healing Common Ailments

Emmett Lokey

the actions taken outside of their direct purview. Regardless, there are zero scenarios where the original author or the Publisher can be deemed liable in any fashion for any damages or hardships that may result from any of the information discussed herein.

Additionally, the information in the following pages is intended only for informational purposes and should thus be thought of as universal. As befitting its nature, it is presented without assurance regarding its prolonged validity or interim quality. Trademarks that are mentioned are done without written consent and can in no way be considered an endorsement from the trademark holder.

CHAPTER 1

HISTORY AND INTRODUCTION

Very early in humanity, we find biblical references: "And God said, behold, I gave you all the herbs with seeds On earth. "(Genesis 1:29)

There was one herb an integral part of all life, people, animals, and vegetables since the beginning of the era. Herbal history is not simple. It was involved excursions to the realm of evolution. It takes into account changing factors affecting religious development practice in different countries of the world. There's a problem in myths and history. Can be said to have pioneered the modern science of medicine and chemistry, especially organic chemistry. Understanding natural alchemy derived from the study of herbs and herbal products leads us to a more accurate assessment of aesthetic impact in anthropology.

Mysticism is the pursuit of learning and understanding nature, the original cause, the universal spirit, the use of creativity all that humanity is an integral part. Herbal research and Herbal products provide access to relevant knowledge, demonstration of the universality of creation.

As philosopher Hegel "All knowledge is one. If we can know everything about one thing, we know everything."

The dictionary defines herbs as "woodless seed plants." Tissue that dies entirely or on the ground after flowering; "A herb that has evaluated for its medicinal properties, sweet aroma, and taste. "

Relics and other evidence before the story begins evidence discovered by archaeologists and researchers indicates that herbs and herbal products played an essential role in the lives of individuals and communities of those who developed the use of God-given features of creativity.

From legends and early records, we know that herbs and herbs the product has used as incense. In many cases, under the leadership of old priests, beyond the power of tribal leaders, sweet-smelling substances were burned to soothe the gods. Its growing awareness soon saw that herbal products from which frankincense has made had both healing properties and pleasant scents and that the priest became a "medicine man" and a religious leader of the people. Convinced her. From this primitive beginning, the modern science of healing has evolved.

Probably the oldest genuine record related to use of herbs, herbal products, and related ingredients as perfumes. Medical purpose and perfume measurement found to record hieroglyphs of western royal tombs and temples Nile riverbank near the ancient city of Tevez Egypt. These tombs are estimated to have been built thousands of years before the Christian era. In these records, honey is mentioned as a portion of food and because of its healing properties. This knowledge about the use of herbs and herbal products

In a variety of ways, such as records of temples and tombs Pharaoh's land did not occur naturally this special time. So it is logical to conclude that it has established practice and application of many properties of herbs their derivatives, which can be called herbal products, can trace their traces.

Beginning, through legends and folklore, and since in many countries the development and beginning of civilization. Understanding this, Herbal studies are an excursion into the natural arena alchemy.

Since the legendary era, long before the earliest records are considered historical, few relics showing the development of aesthetic sentiment among Homo sapiens representatives have been found. The Neanderthals and their predecessors were probably busy protecting themselves from natural enemies and could not think of anything but brute force against the dangers of being. However, in cave paintings and sculptures originating from the Cromagnon era, certain characters can be interpreted as burning incense and using products with sweet scents of herbs.

Some esoteric researchers say Cro-Magnons they may have been descendants of Atlantis survivors explain the sudden increase in aesthetic practice man. One factor in favor of faith is the earliest historical evidence, inhabitants of surrounding territories Mediterranean-Carthage, North Africans, Egyptians, Arabs, Israelis, Phoenicians, Greeksand the Romans-were the first registered users of herbal products such as incense, perfume, and medicine. The use of fragrances, and the use of herbal products for pharmacological purposes and the healing arts, is a short step to their use as food, assuming decorating food to make it more delicious is logical. There is no concrete evidence, but even before the so-called civilizations began, herbal products may have instinctively used as food.

From the beginning, at every stage of human existence discover the complexity of modern life that herbs and herbal products have was essential in the economy of life.

Herbs and herbal products are not the same. Inside the facility the world's nature is complex, organized and systematic controlled alchemy and chemistry lab. Chlorophyll, the green pigment of plants, in the alchemical process of photosynthesis, that means the chemical combination of oxygen in the air the motivation of light energy, water from the ground forms starch and cellulose. It is a fundamental component of all plant and animal tissues.

Each species of plant variety is specific chemical element or compound to be stored its cells, together with starch and cellulose. The term herbal product you can refer to these individually saved connections. Whether the plant has developed woody tissue as its general partmetabolism. HERBALISM's extensive research has inspection of herbal products related to a living economy and for human happiness.

In addition to using plants as food for everyone land on earth when people grow into consciousness herbs and plant products have baked to worship God incense and offerings to pagan gods. From all countries ancient Egypt was arguably the first to expand this practice incorporating many of the related features we have a famous example of today "Early science and art of perfume and perfume making it started in ancient Egypt. Egyptians because it is so closely related to the new priesthood- the choice of delighting or soothing the gods, we first used herbal products as a medicine to relieve pain and cure disease. The earliest Chinese records explain the use of incense and smell oriental material. It was ceremonial and religious ceremony, wedding, funeral. However, hieroglyphic records of early Egyptian culture have provided the only ongoing expression of the development of the so-called "smell industry" and its continuous growth to the present universal multi-billion-dollar scale.

Pharaoh's land is more than just establishing its hieroglyphs physical evidence to confirm written or detailed descriptions, as well as records that have raised historian interest. In that case Pharaoh Tutankhamen's tomb was discovered late and found in 1922, the treasures of the burial chamber undoubtedly had vessels designed for frankincense and perfume. Of course, the scent had evaporated more than 3,000 years after the mummy has placed, but the smell remained in the container as unmistakable evidence of the material once contained.

From records and evidence of fact, the "scent of heaven" of perfume was somehow related to hope immortal, and perhaps that's the reason for aromas and other herbs the product has always filled with mummies. Herbal products also used in the mummification process. Biochemical studies have shown that certain chemical elements have required to complete human metabolism. These elements must be present in the food we eat in a form that is available for assimilation.

Chemical analysis shows honey contains mineral elements often in Essen, it is short. Aluminum, calcium, chlorine, copper, iron, Manganese, magnesium, phosphorus, potassium, silicon, sodium, all or some of them may be missing on average in "processed" foods the average family purchases on the market today have included in honey. Some soils may not contain certain elements required by plants, but the amount of each component may be different because it contains traces of honey, which has needed for everyone's metabolism.

Legends and folklore combine honey and another product. While apple cider vinegar is not always a herbal product, and it is beneficial the effects are closely related to them and compliment them of honey in relieving many diseases that can be caused by defects worth mentioning. Some people told glass of water contains a mixture of honey and apple cider vinegar

Minerals, especially potassium to promote physical health and restful sleep.

Honey has a proven bactericidal property. Folklore of many nationalities from the countryside of New England, Canada, Midwest, early French and Spanish descendants

New Orleans, Louisiana, Mississippi, Alabama, California, Pioneer North Pacific countries mentioned beneficial properties many common diseases, especially airway discomfort overload.

Received some reports on honey use applies to skin infections. According to the statement, the result is it was wonderful. Infection disappeared within two days the healing has completed in a week. In addition to using food, honey has recognized in ancient Egypt and the Mediterranean for medicinal properties. Over the centuries, many people have used honey for its healing properties.

Early days when Egypt expanded its power become a known world leader that reflects this impact offerings to Phoenician gods. Then came Carthage and Greece, and finally Rome. The similarities in the practice of using herbal products, both as a sacrifice to their gods and in other ways, are becoming increasingly apparent. A whole series of conquests and defeats known in history. The hegemony struggle continued in the Pnick War. The Latin name of the Phoenicians was POENI, hence the name pnick. From 264 BC until the Carthage ultimately defeated Publius Cornelius ScipioÆmilianus in 146 BC. Disrupted city-states continued to exert their influence in countries around the Mediterranean. The remains of Carthage became the Roman province, and Roman customs confirmed the use of herbal products. Attempts to restore the city lasted until 29 BC. It failed when Emperor Augustus Caesar, the successor to Julius Caesar, rebuilt and became one of the most famous cities in the Roman

Empire. That time to its destruction by the Arabs in 698, the use of herbal products to personalize and beautify the food took precedence over the choices offered to the gods.

Discovery and development the use of musks in incense and perfumes is due to this

Chinese. Musks are not primarily herbal products, can not be classified by herbs, its use has been for centuries closely related to herbal products that do not mention it in harmony with the scope of this work.

But there are good examples of real herbs, Even before the age of Confucius, it features a Chinese image that dates back more than 2000 years. Botanically speaking, this herb belongs to the arachnid family, which has characteristics similar to the fruit fly family, except that the fruit is a monolithic termite.

Cherry-A soft, fleshy fruit that surrounds a hard-shelled stone or seed. This plant family contains more than 50 genera. These are alarias represented by many species, including Spikenard and Sarsaparillas. Hedera is an example of ivy. Echinopanax, "The Devil's Club". Panax of ginseng.Panax contains most two specific herbs excellent with their claimed properties and features and uses. The native plant in China is Panax Shenzhen, a real herb that is often 2-3 feet tall. There are tiny green flowers, crimson fruit, intricate leaves consisting of five leaves, and things like five-leaf ivy. But most important is the root. American species Panax quinquefolia is little different from that Asian varieties and their roots are identical in production and use. Individual books attributed to Confucius praised its roots this herb for her healing power. Confucius its use by the Chinese dates back to 500 years ago it is probably hundreds of years. Still used in Chinese medicine. The old way of preparing a route for use was a secret process.

Only Chinese pharmacists know. The unbroken or complete route broken and healed to an apparent translucency by this secret process. Today, such roots can bring hundreds of dollars in the Chinese market, multiples of the price of international gold. Prepared in this way, wrapped in fine silk and put in small ones Jewellery boxes, roots were considered a suitable gift to a powerful Chinese enhancer. For centuries, ginseng has been considered a "fountain of youth" for plants and is particularly useful as an aphrodisiac to restore vitality and vitality to the elderly. The Chinese believe that it extends their lifespan. Many great treatments have been attributed to this root by Orientals. Probably an enterprising Yankee of the 18th century the captain of the Oriental Trade has an idea. He knew it as well. The plant species grew up in his New England house, and he gave birth Hundreds of pounds of roots with him on the next trip. The reaction was enormous, and Yankee property has created. He returned the rich. Today there are millions of people in the southeast Asia wants to buy more than we can produce. Prices are still up pharmacologist.

No useful properties of the root have yet been discovered and have not listed in the United States Pharmacopeia. It takes 5 to 8 years to grow to a salable size. Due to very high prices and rising prices, some US farmers have included ginseng in their harvest schedules quite extensively. Ginseng root taste somewhat uncomfortable. It has a faint bittersweet scent reminiscent of liquorice aftertaste. Chinese believe that tea made from ginseng root has healed Tuberculosis treats or prevents many other diseases physical and mental fatigue. Cannot be classified as "fashion."

Long history as a classic and its steady increasing demand. No records found demonstrating the use of ginseng powder root the mixture of herbs as incense. it's fun right experiments with adding ginseng root, powder or dried leaves burn fruits to other plant matter and use the mix as incense investigate any apparent effects.

Archaeologist and anthropologist still trying to solve parent-child issues

Indian. Many theories have developed. Some authorities say red people in North America descendants of the original hill builder, its artefacts

Stand out along the Ohio River valley. Origin of The hill builder himself is an unresolved secret, such as the question "What happened to them?"

It is now generally accepted that humans (Homo sapiens) were not the consequence of another act of creation: that it evolved from a more straightforward form of animal life. Zoologically speaking, the closest relative of humans-humanity Monkeys are all found in Europe, Asia and Africa. Pratilinsal South and Central America are more biologically far from humans. More than in the Old World, and they didn't have them it was Indian ancestry. Seems ethnic make sure Indians are from a human race or tribe creatures that later came to the United States from Eurasia and Australia developed the characteristics of Homo Sapiens. No missing link the skeleton has found in the United States to date. There is from archaeological research, humans presence in North America 11,000 or 12,000 years ago. From where did he come, and how did he go to North America?

History and welfare if there is a problem Humanity imagines that many beautiful hearts are starting to make suggestions solution. Evidence is in geology, palaeontology, zoology, Botany, archaeology, ethnology, and even religion. From the mass of collected data, specific theories evolve, none you can prove 100% accuracy.

Probably the most common theory is that Indians came to North America from Asia (Siberia) via Bering Road during the last ice depression in the Pleistocene.

Geological studies show that overpasses are likely to be interconnected Asia and Alaska probably several times in thousands of years when a continental glacier disappears. Old Indian. When they came to Alaska this way, they probably didn't come suddenly

Immigration rush. They cannot know under any circumstances waiting for them in the south and east. Geologist, The continental ice cap was probably hundreds of meters thick. To tell the widespread presence of Indians in North America the consequences of this infiltration alone will be very suspicious.

Another theory put forward by some authorities is that Indians the descendants of Southwest, Mexico and Central America. An ancestor of the South Pacific. The similarity between physical characteristics and habits shows the truth of this assumption. It is

Considering certain factors in Old Indian life, many open question. How did you get here? at that time original Settlement, Shipping and Cruise in North America

It was probably impossible to be far away from the South Sea islands. Some philosophical thinkers "Lost Atlantic and Lemuria" form an overpass

From Africa to Latin America these include Easter Island, Hawaii and the Marquesas Group. The argument contains only a Ziggurat or Step pyramid. Peru, Bolivia, Central America, Egypt,

MesopotamiaGrotesque statue of Easter Island and Nankai Group. Imagination? Maybe We cannot prove at the moment.

Some religious groups assume that they are Old Indians descendants of the lost tribe of the house of Israel. There is no proof in the Bible to support the idea of mass migration

In the Old Testament, if it was, it was a lot it's too late to explain the broad population of North America. The theory of "continental migration" has proposed to take this into account due to the assumption that the continent used to be where the sea once existed

Today. According to this belief, North and South America connected to Europe and Africa millions of years ago, solid ground surface. The old name of this "continent."

Gondwanaland. Then, when the earth cools and shrinks, appeared, and the land on the ground separated and drifted. Difficulty the behaviour had zoologically performed long before a person developed. But, regardless of their origin, they came to Old Indians

At least 11,000 inhabitants in South and South America, probably more than 20,000 years before the so-called discovery 1492 Western Columbus continent. Changes in that habit and before that time the general economy of life was slow and the problem of adaptation to the environment. Reconstructed image explain the truth that geography is a parent in life at this point of history.

Legends and history unite into almost amazing stories magic effect and healing properties Indian herbal blend, tea, envelope and its medicine and a tremendous healing effect. Ritual in all tribes and tribal happiness was the direct responsibility of the medical scientist and his assistant. In most cases, he had more real power

boss. From an extensive study of Indian folklore, legends and history from different tribes in North America and many visits India reservations and talks with the elderly

General conclusions have drawn for young people. During exercise and old and modern customs were somewhat different basic pattern due to genetic and ecological differences

It seems to penetrate the life of both Old Indians and Old Indians their descendants. This pattern has expressed by looking at two things.Related factors.

First, regardless of its origin and subsequent northern settlements Americans and Indians were basically "mysterious". That is, they have their beliefs, habits, and

ceremony. All tribes had many festivals. Every day, from simple rituals to rituals that last several days. But all rituals were based on the perception of high power and the universality of great medicine and great spirit of course, different tribes had their best names he who exerted this power and the minds below.

The second factor is in all ceremonies and herbs, Herbal products have used to demonstrate the emotions drawn by special events have celebrated. Properties of the herbs used related to the desired effect. Before white comes, lofty and beautiful

An Indian philosophy called "Progress." "Noble Redman" was not just a phrase. Research is done by American Museum of Natural History, Smithsonian Institution,

United States Department of Agriculture and individuals Archaeologists and ethnologists have revived ancient legends and folk tales of early North American residents. Taking these reports into account necessarily leads to a natural the conclusion that they share a common foundation the similarity of origin. I can explain the differences between the tribes by recognizing the effects of climate and the environment

Explain the differences in story details from the old tribal man around the campfire at night. Key facts in every story, the Supreme God, the Great Spirit, Excellent medicine, God, or the name they assigned to himMighty ruler, this power always appeared

Nature-by growing plants and because animals eat plants. All creatures can participate in this power. Many examples show this fact. There were some in all strains where corn was grown ceremonies including tree-planting festivals, the appearance of the first ear, the beginning of harvest grain storage for future livelihoods. Shaman or medicine

The man (called "Sakem" in some tribes) presided over them in some cases, they lasted several days. Probably the most Algonquins and Algonquins performed the elaborate ceremony East and Northeast Iroquois. There were three powerful Indian nations in the east and northeast. The most populous were the Algonquins, but they were not very wealthy -Five tribes organized as the Iroquois Federation: Oneidas, Mohawks, Senecas, Onondagas, Cayugas. This club it has based on blood relationships. Among them they were peaceful in their home life. Your village was permanent Each "lodge" had its characteristics, where tribal women lived Grew corn, beans, pumpkins, pumpkins and gourds and other herbs that made up most of their food. That is community life. Early French missionaries are new the country, shortly after 1600, they discovered the life of this closely related village, Women were the dominant provider longhouse

The property of women who were builders and farmers Labour force. Men were allowed to live with them as long as they were acted. Harvest of corn and other herbs and tobacco unusually the property of the community.

HISTORY OF THE USE OF TRADITIONAL CHINESE MEDICINE

By definition, the "traditional" method of herbal medicine means important historical use. It is true for many products available as "traditional Chinese medicine." In many under developing and well-developed countries, a large proportion of the population depends on traditional practitioners, arming them with medicinal plants to ensure the health nursing needs. Although modern medicine can exist with such conventional medicine Herbal medicines are often becoming historical and popular Cultural reasons. Such products have marketed on a larger scale, especially in developed countries.

In this modern environment, ingredients have sometimes sold for applications never considered in the original traditional healing system surfaced. Examples are the use of ephedra (= Ma huang) for weight loss or exercise. Improved performance (Shaw, 1998). Chinese medicine is available in some countries it is subject to strict manufacturing standards and does not apply everywhere. In Germany for example, if herbal products have sold as "phytomedicine," they will same efficacy, safety, and quality standards as other drugs. In the United States in contrast, most herbal products on the market are sold and regulated as diet products product categories without additional product pre-approval based on any of these criteria.

The role of Chinese herbal medicine in traditional healing pharmacological treatment of the disease began long ago with the use of herbs (Schulz et al., 2001). Folk remedies around the world Herbs as part of the tradition. Some of these traditions had briefly described below. Provides some examples of the number of critical healing practices around the world Herbs used for this purpose.

CHINESE HERBAL MEDICINE

Chinese medicine has been used by the Chinese since ancient times. Animal and mineral ingredients have used, but this is the primary treatment it is a plant. Of the more than 12,000 times used by traditional healers, about 500 shared use (Li, 2000). Plant products have used after they have processed.

It may include, for example, roasting or dipping with vinegar or wine. Clinically

In fact, after a traditional diagnosis, complex prescriptions can be prescribed often a personalized treatment.Traditional Chinese medicine is still widely used in China. More than half of the population regularly uses the most common conventional treatments in rural areas. There are about 5,000 traditional treatments in China. They make up about one-fifth of the total Chinese pharmaceutical market (Li, 2000).

JAPANESE TRADITIONAL MEDICINE

Many herbal remedies have found a way from China to the Japanese system traditional healing. Herbs native to Japan had classified in the first pharmacopeia Japanese traditional medicine in the 9th century (Saito, 2000).

INDIAN TRADITIONAL MEDICINE

Ayurveda is a medical system mainly implemented in India, almost 5,000 years. Includes diet and herbal remedies while stressing the body mind and soul in the prevention and treatment of disease (Morgan, 2002).

Introduction of traditional Chinese medicine in Europe, the United States, and the United States other developed countries. The desire to gain the wisdom of conventional healing systems have aroused interest in Chinese herbal medicine, especially in Europe and the north (Tyler, 2000).

In the United States, where herbal products have incorporated into so-called "alternatives." A "complementary", "global", or "integrated" medical system.

In the other half of the 20th century, interest in self-care increased.

The surge in popularity of traditional healing methods, including using Herbal remedies, this is especially true in the United States. Consumers reported positive attitude to these products. They believe that their origin is more "natural" than "composite" and that such products tend to do so considered safer than drugs and part of a healthy lifestyle, To avoid unnecessary contact with traditional "Western" medicine.

Centuries of use in traditional environments serve as evidence that certain herbal ingredients are active or safe, but need to address a variety of issues elements have incorporated into modern customs. One problem is that the ingredients used for symptomatic treatment in traditional healing have now used in well-developed countries as part of health promotion or illness. Prevention strategies; therefore, acute treatment has replaced by chronic exposure (e.g., Herbal products for weight loss, Allison et al. , 2001). It means a statement"Thousands of years of evidence that a product is safe."The product is currently in use. It does not explicitly mean that the ingredients are not safe. In other words, security is unacceptable in modern times.

The second problem is that efficacy and effectiveness have poorly demonstrated in modern scientific research. There is an evidence-based approach to this problem

Recently implemented, the results are for most herbal products, to be convinced of knowledge, you need to fill a significant gap in knowledge their effectiveness.

One of the most challenging problems when translating traditional herbs Traditional "Western" medicine practice is the personalization of prescriptions tt contains some herbs and other ingredients. There is little incentive to standardize products for the mass market when aiming to provide custom recipes. For smallholders and traditionally trained herbalists, standardization means understanding growing conditions, harvest times, and methods

Reliable (even in small quantities) by material extraction or other preparation active ingredients have provided to people. To significant manufacturers and dealers standardization relates to quantities sold in supermarkets or health food stores for industrial production under defined conditions, using so-called ethical manufacturing

practices similar to drugs (GMP) (Food & Drug Administration, 2002) production.

In the United States, herbal products had made on a small and large scale market content and quality can vary widely. US regulations do not yet require dietary supplement manufacturers to comply with them quality has not guaranteed due to standard manufacturing practices.That the report discourages the public from looking at products not found on store shelves consistently includes the components or amounts listed on the label.

For frequently used herbal products, proof of efficacy has based on traditional use, experiences, clinical trials, uncontrolled trials, and randomized, double-blind, placebo-controlled trials. But in most cases, it is missing a systematic clinical trial to support the claim. The safety of some herbal ingredients has partially questioned recently. Moreover, based on the identification of adverse events related to their use for evidence of clinically relevant interactions between herbs and prescription drugs. Adverse events (stroke, heart attack, abnormal heart rate, hepatotoxicity, stroke, Psychoses and Death) Weight loss, related to the use of ephedra for bodybuilding common effects and increased energy in Europe, or kava (aka kava) treat anxiety, tension, insomnia, pain, and muscle more and more in Canada for example, tensions have led some countries to adopt or restrict regulations ban on these products (Health Canada Online, 2002a, b, etc.). Just a few herbs general use has suspected of causing cancer. Use of traditional Chinese medicine in developed countries.

ORIGIN, TYPE, AND PLANT DATA

The components of plants and their secondary metabolites are: In individual systems of modern "Western" and traditional medicine, Sources of essential pharmaceuticals such as atropine, codeine, digoxin, morphine, quinine vincristine.

Herbal medicine use in developed countries has increased significantly in the latter countries half of the 20th century. Monographs of selected herbs are available in a range

European Scientific Cooperative for Phytotherapy, German Commission E, and the World Health Organization (WHO, 1999). For example, in the WHO monograph, the herbs themselves number of criteria (including synonyms and native names) and parts of herbs the commonly used geographic distribution is herbs (including gross and microscopic examinations and purity checks), active principles (if known), drug forms and dosages, medical uses, pharmacology, contraindications and side effects. Other resources that provide more information on the herbal products currently in use are a comprehensive database of natural medicines (Jellin, 2002) and NAPRALERT (NAtural PRoducts ALERT) (2001). Information about other available databases has published by Bhat (1995).

MEDICAL USES, BENEFICIAL EFFECTS AND ACTIVE INGREDIENTS

In some cases, the active parts of herbal products had separated, have been characterized and their mechanism of action is understood (eg, ephedrine alkaloids) some types of ephedra). However, for most people, almost everyone natural products on the market, such information is incomplete or unavailable. That is mainly due to the complexity of herb and plant preparation. There is no pure connection. It is also a function of the traditionally believed that the combination of synergistic effects of multiple active ingredients is responsible for some herbal supplements for those beneficial effects.Recognition, control, regulation, usage

WHO GUIDELINES FOR HERBAL MEDICINES

In 1992, the WHO Western Pacific Regional Office invited an expert group develop standards and general principles to guide research on herbal evaluation pharmaceuticals (WHO, 1993). This group recognized the importance of Chinese medicine the health of many people around the world says, "Some people have Chinese medicine. Although endured scientific tests, others have used for protection for traditional reasons, restore or improve health. Most herbal medicines still need to be scientifically investigated. Experience gained from many years of traditional use,

Ignored. There is no evidence to back up with a general scientific approach answers questions about the safety and efficacy of most herbal medicines currently used. Others support reasonable use and further development of herbal medicines proper scientific research of these products and therefore such research. "

Previously reported as Matricaria chamomilla (WHO, 1999) Chinese medicine, evaluation of Chinese medicine research, guidelines for quality specifications of plant materials and preparations, and pharmacodynamics and general pharmacological and toxicity studies of herbal medicines herbal medicine.

WHO has also published guidelines for the evaluation of herbal medicines (WHO, 1996). These guidelines have defined essential criteria for assessing quality, safety, and security efficacy of herbal medication to support national regulatory authorities documentation, submission, and documents related to such products. It has recommended considering such an assessment. A description of long-term use (at least for decades) in the country, Medical and pharmaceutical literature or similar sources or documents from knowledge and approval of the use of Chinese medicine similar products. There are long-term and apparent uses of the substance, Usually proves its safety and naturally checks for potential toxicity the resulting material may reveal problems that were not previously suspected. Regulators also have the authority to promptly respond to new information on toxicity by revoking or restricting the license of registered products containing suspicious substances, or by reclassifying substances and limiting their use to pharmaceuticals Recommended that recipe. Guidelines emphasized the need to evaluate the efficacy, including effectiveness determination of the pharmacological and clinical effects of the active substance label with a quantitative list of active ingredients, dosages, and contraindications. Combination products plant ingredients used in combination had widely used in Europe often, evaluations have made according to specific guidelines. Herbal combination Homeopathic ingredients are present in some countries. Your rating will last faster strict criteria, usually the requirements for a "complete" application process. Herbal combination ingredients and vitamins are available in many countries.

ESCOP AND WHO MONOGRAPHS

European Plant Scientific Therapy Cooperative (ESCOP) (see Awang, 1997) or WHO monographs have used as summaries of data published in the many Member States.

Many regulators consider it a useful document to clarify the effectiveness and security. European Commission (EC), EMEA (European Evaluation Agency) the Executive Director and the EMEA Board established the EMEA Ad Hoc Group in 1997. This working group has comprised of representatives of Member States (mainly health authorities) and EU representatives. European Parliament, EC, and European Pharmacopoeia. walking group review the criteria to demonstrate quality, preclinical safety, and clinical safety effectiveness of listed herbal medicines in marketing approval applications in Council guidelines. Working Group proposes requirements for non-clinical trials of herbal medicines based on the EC Guide Draft for the Elderly a substance with a long history (EMEA, 2000). The group also has it the appropriate role of scientific monograph created by WHO and ESCOP.

SIMPLIFIED PROOF OF VALIDITY

In addition to fully approved herbal medicines, many traditional herbal medicines are present in the many Member States. State authorities for these products as a general rule, check security and ensure an appropriate level of quality. To demonstrate the effect, requirements levels are simplified because they may adjust for years of experience. For example, there are specific uncomplicated steps Austria, Belgium, France, Germany. Most other countries in the EU do not use this strategy.

FURTHER DEVELOPED PRODUCTS

Herbal medicines with different indications proposed or modified compared to traditional forms (such as highly processed or special ones extract), in most cases, requires a full license, and efficacy must clinically have proven in the study. Such products have not used in some countries.

CHAPTER 2

SOME USEFUL HERBS

ALOE VERA

Herbal aloe vera

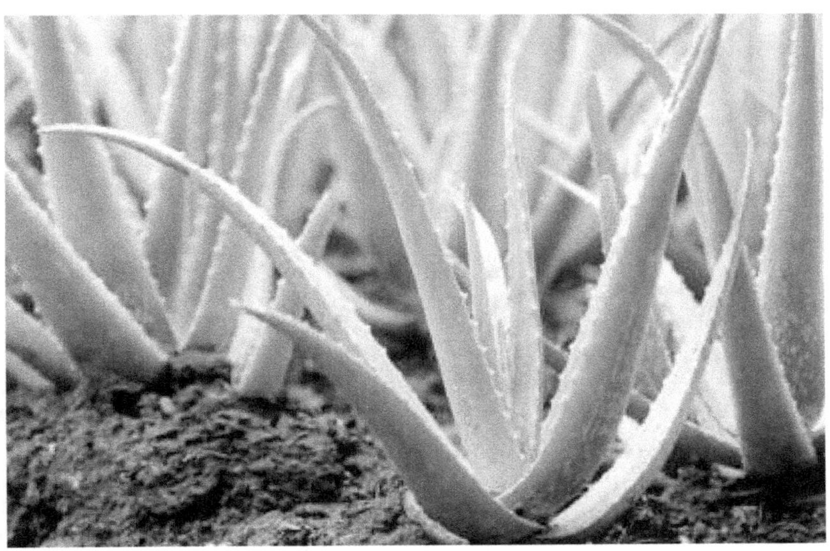

Aloe vera plants are at the top of the list of herbs and their uses. Aloe plants are rich in medicinal properties and have used for this reason for centuries. Aloe plants are relatively easy to grow once they have established. No need to water daily or weekly. It makes Aloe plants perfect for those who are out and about to forget to water.

Important medical applications

Burns

psoriasis

Diabetes

Colitis

Support the immune system

Anti-inflammatory

Skin toner

Wound healer

Aloe gel against burns

Aloe gel for burn

The most common use of aloe should be in the treatment of burns, wounds, and skin disorders. Moreover, to be easy to grow aloe plants, it is an excellent choice for your herbal first aid kit. The real magic of aloe vera lies in the leaf gel. That is needed to extract it to remove the knife and remove the thick skin outside the sheet. What I'm looking for is a transparent inner gel, also called an inner fillet, to fill the leaves. For minor burns, flush the affected area with cold water for about 10 minutes before applying aloe gel. Apply gel several times a day to combat wounds and skin conditions. If you use aloe gel to lower blood sugar, take about one tablespoon a day. (For oral use, apply aloe gel that does not contain aloe.)

Be careful

When using aloe, care must be taken not to apply it to open wounds. Be careful when processing the leaves. As above, use a bright gel piece to keep away from leaking yellow juice. Applying it to the skin is not a big deal, but you should be aware of this yellow juice when taking aloe gel orally. This yellow juice is called Aloin. When received, it acts as a laxative. Prolonged use of Aloin may lead to electrolyte shortages and reliance on normal bowel function.

BASIL

Herb basil

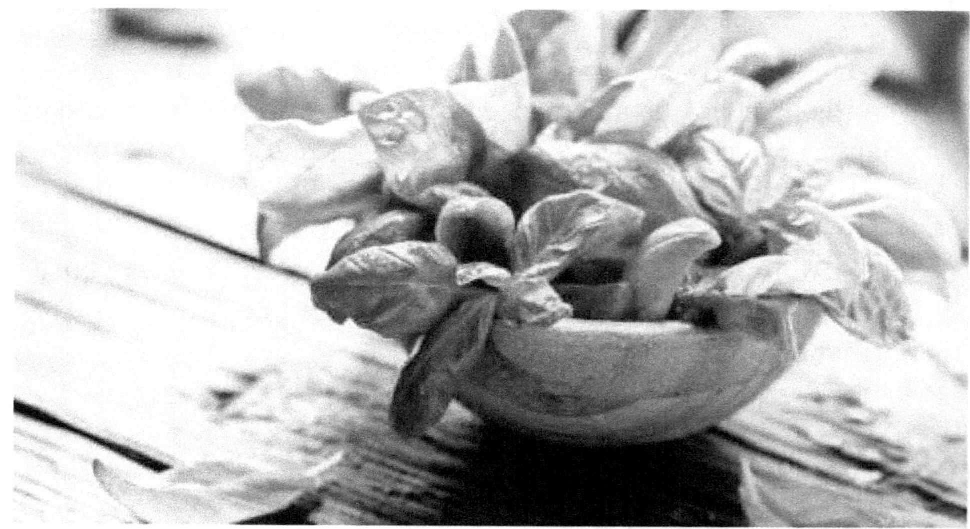

In addition to being a wonderful herb of Basil, it also has a place
as herbal medicine. One of the reasons I really like basil plants is
that they are very easy to grow. You only need to make sure to
water them from time to time. It is also a very aromatic herb
with the scent and taste of licorice. One of the must-do things
you can do with Basil is cloning. That's crazy. It is actually pretty
simple. You have to do is find the plant you want to clone (the
mother plant) and cut it off about 3-4 inches from the top of the
stem. You must cut just above the knot. In this area, leaves
attach to the stem body and new growth takes place. Next,
remove the bottom leaf of the cut and make a stem with 4-6
leaves on top. Then put the cut in a flat water bowl and wait for

the roots to germinate. Next, a new basil clone is planted in the
soil. In order to accelerate root growth, I have found that
applying root hormones and some honey to the end of the stem
is very helpful. As mentioned above, Basil has a status as
Chinese medicine. Let's look at the characteristics of basil plants
that have used.

Important medical applications

antibacterial

Mild sedative

Relieve gas

Bites, bites

Root hormone

Root hormone for cloning

As you can expect from herbs like Basil, it has a rather profound
effect on the digestive system and is perfect for treating
indigestion, gas, and gas. If you use Basil to address these
problems, I recommend taking 2-4 grams orally daily. Basil can
also be used to reduce the effects of insect bites and bites. Just
crush the leaves and you can apply the juice to the affected area.
The fluid can be applied to the skin in the same way so that it is
not bitten or stabbed. It should help to repel insects since Basil
works very well as an insecticide.

MARIGOLD

Herb marigold

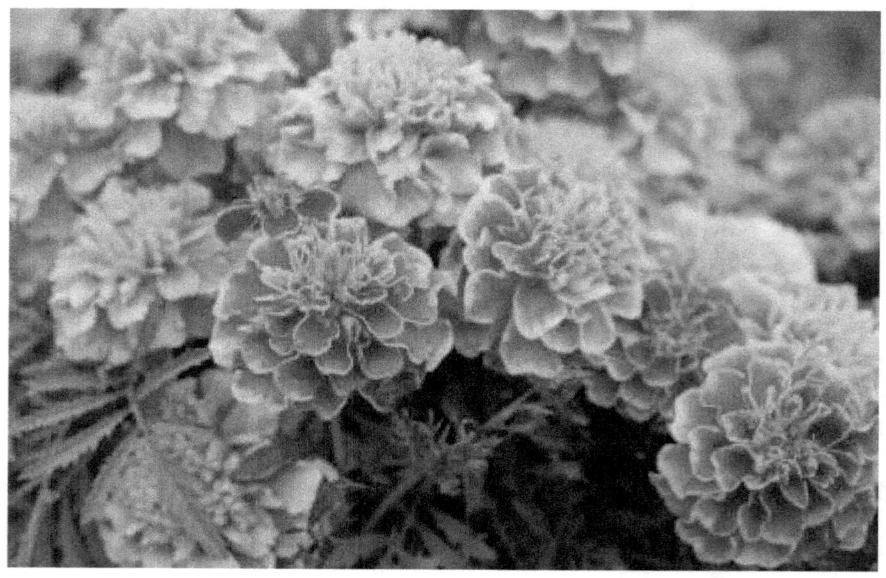

Marigold, also known as the poet's marigold or marigold, is different from the marigold generally found in gardens. In contrast to marigolds, marigolds are edible and have little odor. In medieval Britain, marigold herbs have commonly used in stews, syrups, and loaves of bread. Calendula is also quite easy to start with seeds and can adapt to many growing conditions, making it an ideal herb for growth. Herbs are found in many gardens around the world for subarctic to tropical regions. Next, let's look at the leading medical uses that make Calendula such a popular herb.

Important medical applications

Antifungal

Anti-inflammatory

Wound healer

Antibacterial agent

Blood purifier

Dermatitis

Marigold ointment

Calendar serves

The manufacture of Calendula, lotion, ointment, ointment, and soap is the most common way to use marigold herbs. Calendula has used for centuries to treat some small wound skin diseases and infections. Marigold herbs can also have taken orally to relieve stomach, ulcer, and fever symptoms. In most cases, marigolds have used externally to treat small cuts, burns, insect bites, and more. When applied to treat indigestion, tea, and tinctures made from petals are ideal for treating gastric ulcers and gastrointestinal infections. To alleviate this indigestion it is recommended to take 3-5 grams a day.

Be careful

Avoid using marigolds if you are allergic to plants of the Asteraceae family. You can develop sensitivity to any topical application that can lead to the development of a rash.

CAYENNE PEPPER

Cayenne pepper

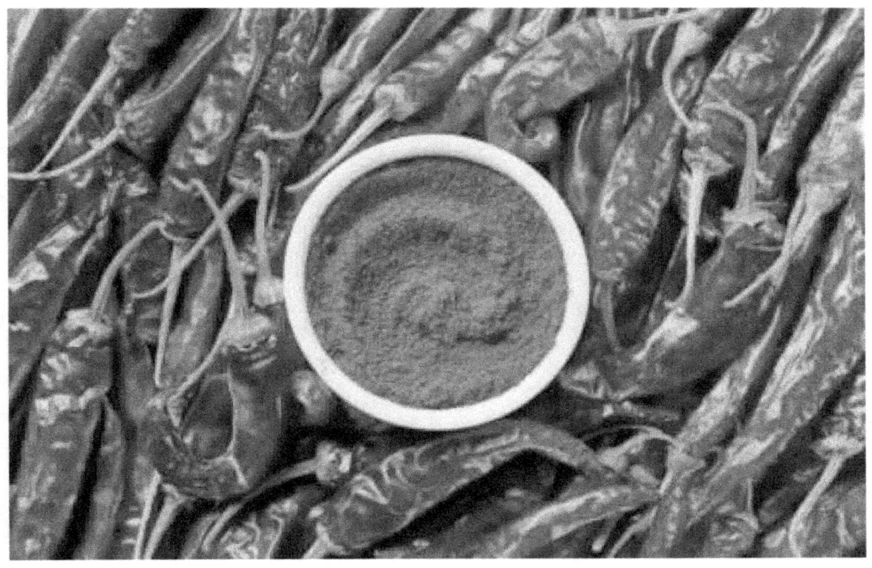

Probably best known for adding spices to dishes. Cayenne
pepper has many to offer as medicinal herbs. Most herbal lists
tend to skip using cayenne pepper for some reason. Apply of
cayenne pepper can be traced back to Aztecs and Mayans.
Usually, they have used for toothache and infections. The main
chemical that has enormous medical benefits is capsaicin. It is
the same chemical that gives the burning sensation when
chewing Jalapeno. If you are interested in tips for growing
peppers, check out the previously published article.

Important medical applications

Preservative

Topical analgesics

Counterstimulus

Stimulant

Relieve gas

arthritis

Neuralgia

Cayenne pepper capsule

Cayenne capsule

Most often, cayenne pepper is used as a cream, lotion, or ointment to treat problems such as arthritis, shingles, and joint and muscle pain associated with fibromyalgia. Ingestion has also has shown to relieve cluster headache pain, improve circulation, and reduce heartburn. For neuralgia, apply a cream containing about 0.075% capsaicin three to four times a day. Applying about 0.025% cream four times a day can also treat the arthritic pain. Cayenne pepper results to work out it, but it only works if you wait patiently. The capsule also contains cayenne pepper, which is a great way to take cayenne pepper orally. In some cases, cayenne pepper is also known to reduce appetite and burn calories but appears to have little effect overall.

Warning

Whenever capsaicin has applied to the skin, it can cause burns, stinging, redness, and even a rash. In most cases, the rash is more irritating than anything and improves with the first few uses. If the rash persists, discontinue use as it may be allergic to capsaicin. Capsaicin never is applied to broken skin. If you work at high concentrations and do not touch your face, remember where to put your gloves. If you are not wearing gloves, you should wash your hands thoroughly before touching your face.

CHAMOMILE

Chamomile

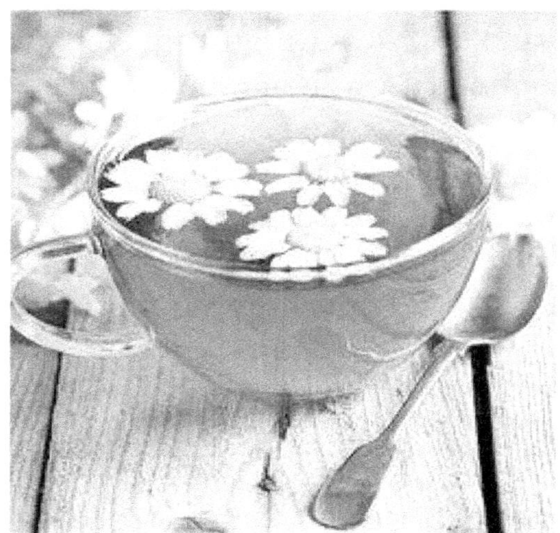

The next herb on the list is chamomile. That is another beautiful herb with a different use. This Spanish name for the grass is Manzanilla, which means "tiny apple." Not surprisingly, the Spanish people gave it this name. If the leaves and petals are damaged, a distinctive apple scent has created. There are two main types of chamomile: German chamomile and Roman or British chamomile. They are all similar in medicinal properties, but the Roman or British model has a more pronounced aroma than the German type. Both are relatively easy to grow from seed. If they are sown by themselves, they will find that they will grow next spring.

Important medical applications

Digestive aid

Colic

Mouth ulcer

eczema

Antiallergic

Anti-inflammatory

Wound healer

Dried chamomile

Dried chamomile

Chamomile is often in the form of tea, making it easy to build a house. Pour boiling water into a teaspoon of dried chamomile. Inject tea for 5-7 minutes. The longer the tea has poured, the stronger the sedative effect. Chamomile capsules have also found, making chamomile quick and easy to use. Making topical chamomile cream is also a great way to relieve the symptoms of eczema. Low doses of hydrocortisone cream have shown to produce the same results as chamomile cream used to treat inflammation.

BE CAREFUL

In rare cases, symptoms of an allergic reaction to chamomile may appear. These are generally people with severe ragweed allergies. In general, chamomile is a very safe herb.

CHICKWEED

Chickweed herb

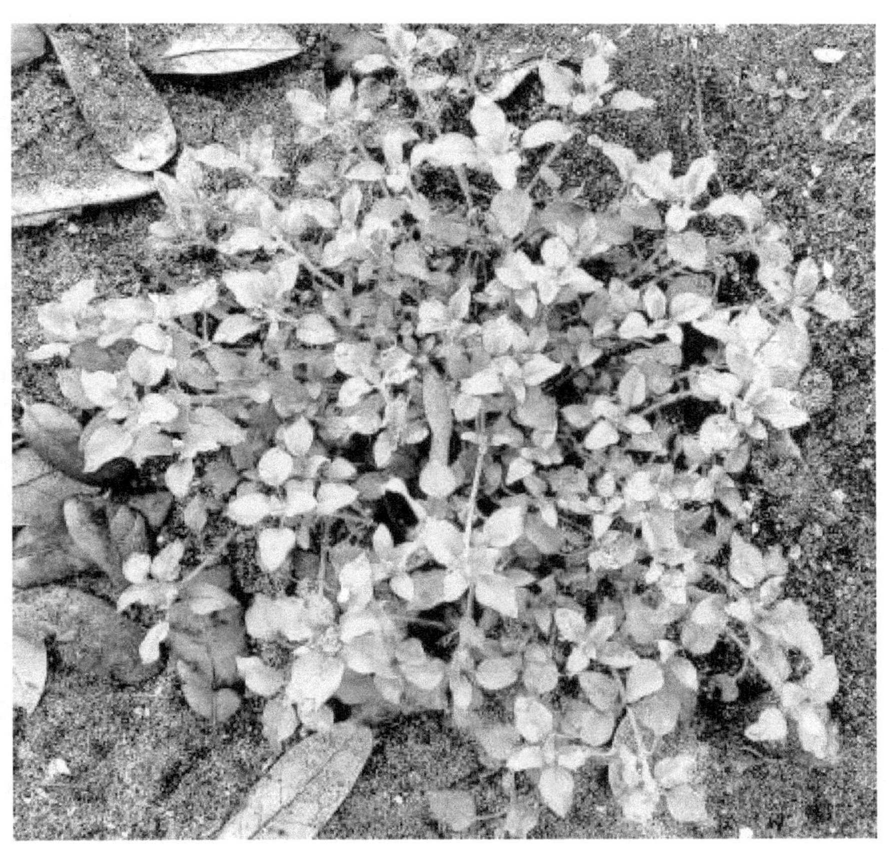

Chickweed is an annual plant found worldwide in temperate and Arctic regions. An exciting feature of chickweed is that it sleeps. At night the leaves break and cover young shoots and buds. Chickweed is also known as a nutritious herb and is perfect for salads. The whole plant has used for both dry and fresh herbs.

Let's look at the main medical uses for which this herb is best known.

Important medical applications

Astringent

Painkillers

Relieve itching

Cooling effect by topical application

Scallop ointment

honey

Chickweed is probably best known for its ability to relieve itching and is often used to treat eczema, nettle rash, and insect bites. By blending olive oil, chickweed, beeswax, and lavender as fragrances, you can make a simple chickweed slave. Finely chop the chickweed and let it dry for about 24 hours. Next, mix the chickpeas and olive oil in equal amounts and mix for about 20 seconds. Next, place the mixture in a metal bowl suspended over another metal bowl with water. Bring the water in the lower pan to a boil. Keep the bottom of the upper bowl away from water. Otherwise, the mixture can get too hot. Stir the mixture frequently before passing through the cheesecloth. Using the same method, melt the beeswax, add the injected oil, stir and mix, then remove. The ointment has placed in a glass for later use.

Be careful

Chickweed can cause an allergic skin reaction. Herbs also contain saponins. Saponins are toxic at high doses. It has recorded that cattle died from too many herbs. You have to eat a few pounds to kill an animal.

CINNAMON

Cinnamon stick

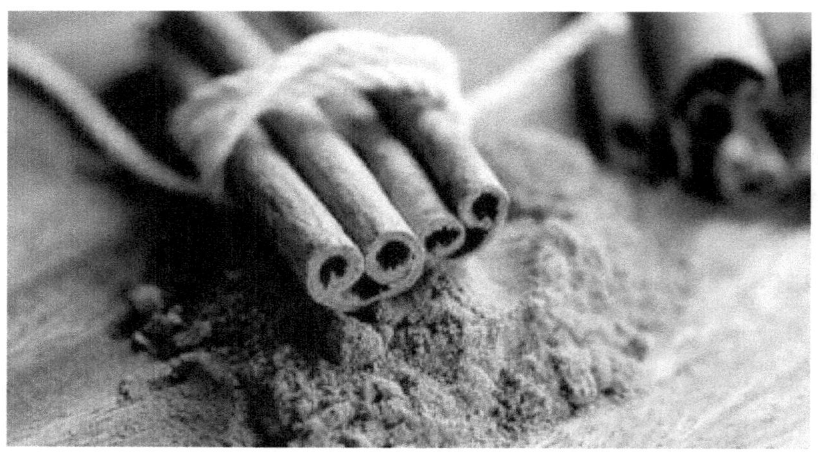

Another well-known spice of kitchen cinnamon is also known for its medicinal properties. It's not a herb, but I think it's essential to list herbs and their uses. Cinnamon has derived from the bark of laurel ancestry. It has been used for centuries and has been a popular product since ancient times. In fact, in Rome in the 1st century AD, cinnamon was 15 times more expensive than silver. The Chinese were probably the first to use cinnamon as a herb and treat fever and diarrhea. Recently, cinnamon has shown to stabilize blood sugar in diabetic patients due to its insulin effect.

Important medical applications

Diabetes

Mild stimulant

Aromatic

Astringent

Antibacterial agent

Relieve gas

cinnamon

Sri Lanka floor room

The primary use of cinnamon is in the treatment of diabetes. Take one teaspoon of cinnamon powder to balance your blood sugar. Cinnamon capsules have found, dosages vary, but generally, 1-6 grams of cinnamon capsules per day is an appropriate amount depending on the distance. An excellent little way to replace cinnamon sugar is to combine freshly ground cinnamon sticks with six teaspoons of stevia. It is excellent for toasts, oatmeal, and fruits.

Be careful

Ground cinnamon is very safe, but volatile oils can cause a rash. Cassia and other types of cinnamon contain small amounts of coumarin. Generally, only high doses of this compound cause blood thinning and liver problems, but this is what you need to know. Even if you are planning a surgery, you should stop using cinnamon at least one week before the procedure, because it helps to thin your blood. Care must have taken to monitor blood sugar levels to avoid unsafe blood pressure drops.

CLOVES

Carnation bud

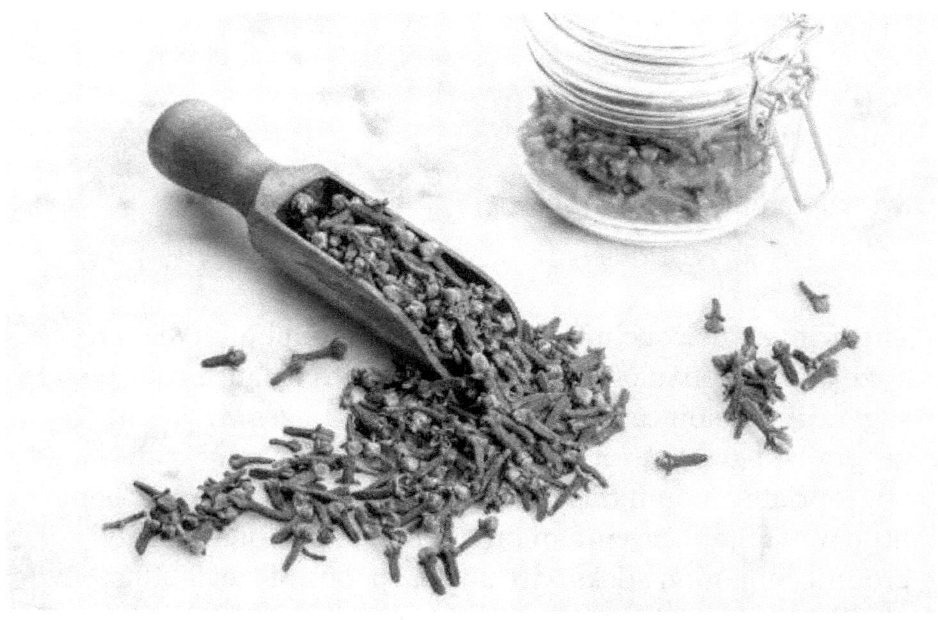

For many, it is surprising that carnations are flower buds. These buds have picked at the right time. The buds turn red before the flowers bloom, making it a great time to harvest cloves. Carnation buds come from evergreen bushes with bright pink flowers and purple berries. Clove plants are perfect for warm and humid areas. The oldest written record of the use of cloves as a medicinal plant dates back to the Han Dynasty in China around 300 BC. Like cinnamon, cloves are a popular spice and used to compete with the value of oil. Let's take a look at what the main medicinal properties of cloves are and how to use this herb.

Important medical applications

Painkillers

Stimulant

Preservative

Antiemetic

Antioxidant

Antibacterial agent

Clove oil

Clove oil

For toothache, apply a drop of clove or clove oil to a cotton ball of a sore tooth. However, use this method with care and do not apply oil to the rubber. In the case of neuralgia, up to 3%, diluted oil can be applied to the skin to treat problems such as shingles. In small amounts, clove powder can help treat nausea, indigestion, and bloating.

Be careful

Do not drink essential oils without careful dilution. In some cases, topical application can cause dermatitis. Use cloves sparingly and be aware of your body's reactions.

COMFREY

Comfrey

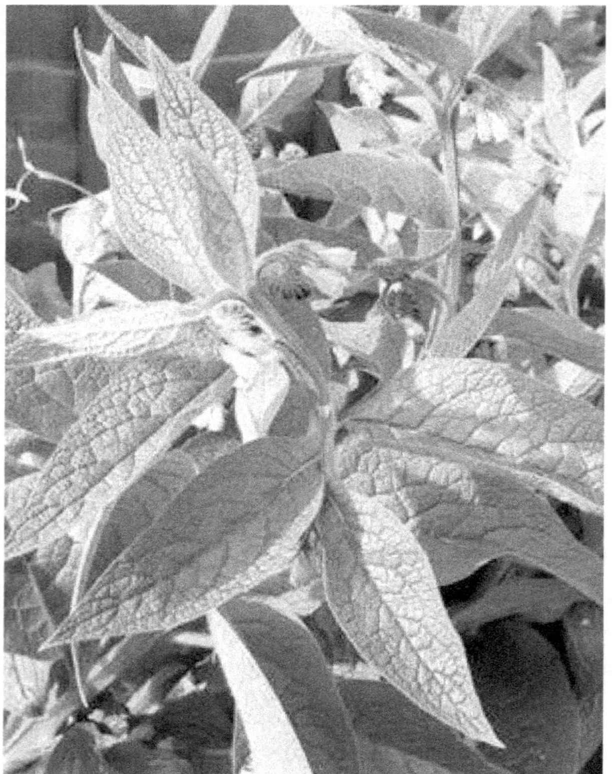

Comfrey used centuries, at least in the days of the ancient Greeks. Comfrey was a common medieval herb that was common in monastery gardens. In the 1700s and 1800s, Comfrey was also a popular herb grown in many gardens in Europe and the United States. However, some point in the late 1970s, research has shown that Comfrey, when taken in the body, can cause severe liver damage, reducing its use and even banning internal use in many countries. However, application to ointments, envelopes, and creams is still considered safe. Comfrey is still growing wild in Central Europe, the eastern United States, and some Western countries.

Important medical applications

Anti-inflammatory

Painkillers

Wound healer

Astringent

HOW TO USE:
Comfrey ointment

COMFREY ointment

Comfrey is perfect today for gels, ointments, creams, salves, or envelopes. Find extracts that remove dangerous alkaloids while relieving pain and maintaining anti-inflammatory properties. Massage one of these methods three or four times a day into your bruises, painful joints, or muscles.

Be careful

As already mentioned that many countries have banned domestic use of Comfrey, we need to warn again not to take Comfrey domestically. The alkaloids it contains can be very harmful to the liver.

DANDELION

Dandelion herb in the bowl

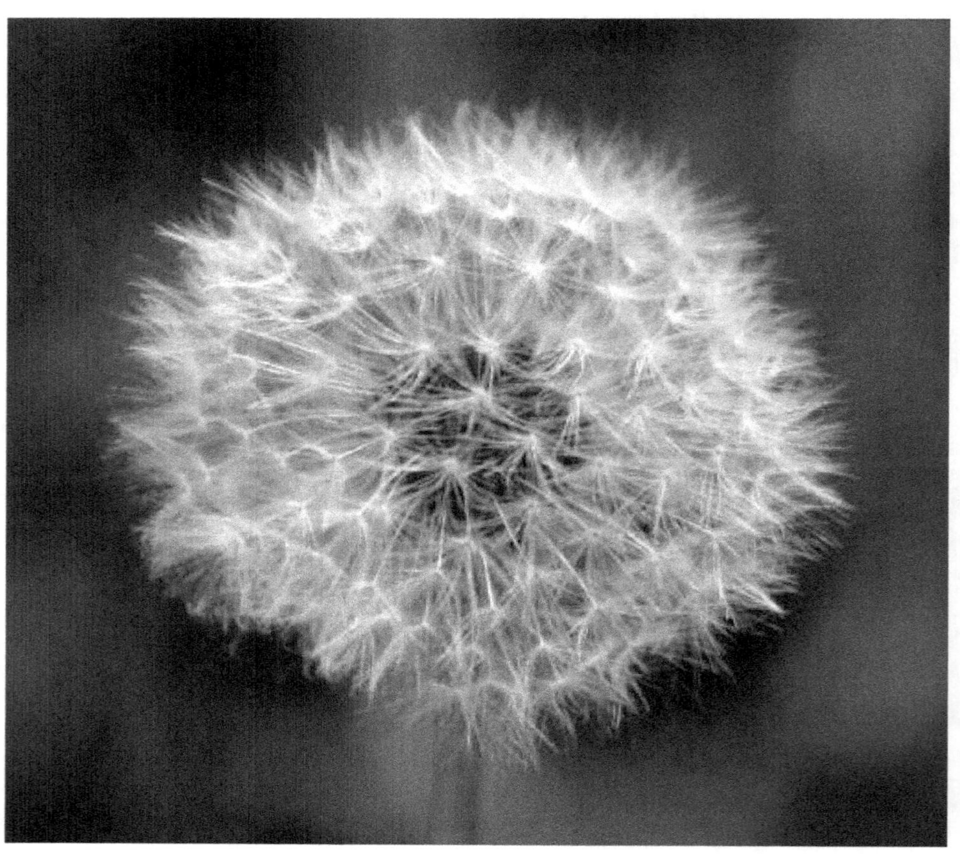

Dandelions have considered weeds because they suffocate the grass across the garden. Dandelion is a wonderful herb and is on the list of herbs because it offers many nutritional benefits and treatments. One great thing about dandelion herbs is that the whole plant has used from flowers to roots. The leaves are perfect for salads. If the flowers are yellow, they can be raw, cooked, or dandelion wine. Even dandelion roots have eaten. Usually, it is roasted and eaten or added to a nice cup of tea. Dandelions are sometimes called urinal beds because of their excellent diuretic effect.

Important medical applications

Diuretic

Liver cleanser

Mild laxative

Kidney cleaner

HOW TO USE:
Dandelion tea

Dandelion tea

As already mentioned, whole dandelion plants have used. Roots have many beneficial medicinal properties on the digestive system, such as the stomach, liver, and pancreas. Dandelion roots helped increase digestive juice secretion and also demonstrated the ability to stabilize blood sugar. Dandelion herb leaves primarily affect the kidneys, helping with water clearance and even weight loss. Dandelion leaves are a common choice for the people who want to lower their blood pressure. Combined with other herbs, it effectively relieves skin problems such as acne, boiling, and eczema.

Be careful

It has generally considered that safe herbal dandelion is harmful
to people who are allergic to ragweed. Also, make sure that the
selected dandelion has not sprayed with herbicides or pesticides.

GARLIC

Garlic herb

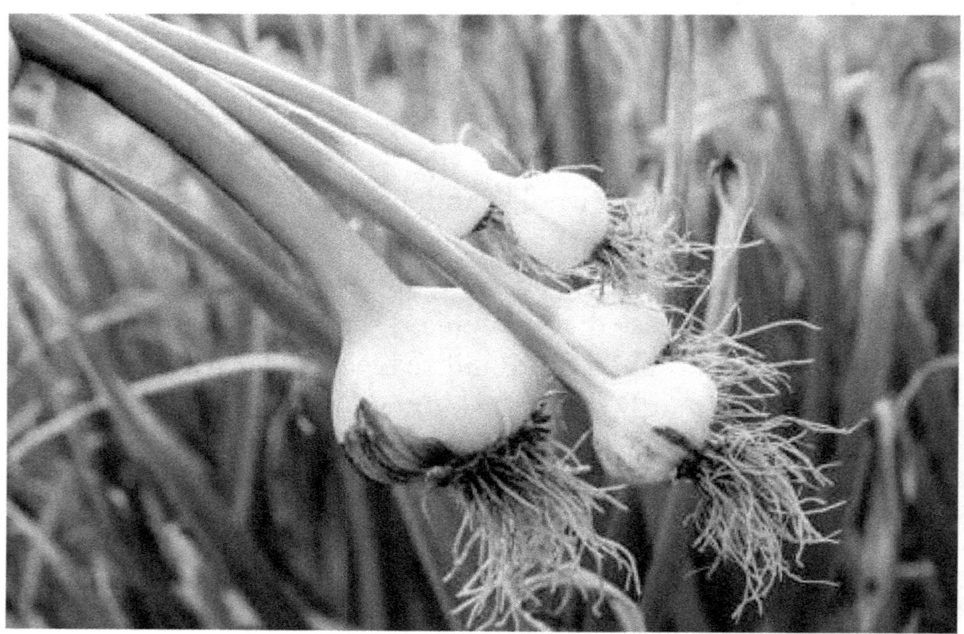

Garlic, a herb commonly used in the kitchen, occupies its place in the herbal list. Garlic has used for thousands of years and is said to increase strength and endurance. The first Olympic athlete used it in Greece, and it could very well make it once of the primary performance-enhancing substances. From vampires to witches, garlic has also used to ward off evil beings with spells and spells. In the Middle Ages, monasteries grew garlic to treat digestive, kidney, and respiratory problems. Allegedly, the Russians ate a lot of garlic during World War II, and some say that this has helped them survive difficult times. Today, garlic has widely used to treat and prevent heart disease, regulate cholesterol, control the high blood pressure, and strengthen the immune system. Garlic overgrows all over the world where home gardens have built. Even indoor garlic works pretty well. You can take the garlic clove and grow the whole garlic plant from that one clove. The next time you're in a supermarket, buy garlic, remove one of the cloves, and plant it on a pointy, moist soil. If you keep watering your cloves regularly, you will soon have beautiful garlic plants. Garlic was probably one of the most critical and often overlooked medicinal herbs on the planet, so it needed to add to the herbal list.

Important medical applications

Antibiotics

Lower blood pressure

Blood diluent

Supports beneficial intestinal flora

For cough and respiratory infections

Antifungal

Lower cholesterol

diarrhea

Heart health

Garlic capsule

Garlic capsule

Raw garlic is the best form of the herb. Cooking garlic destroys many of the ingredients responsible for its medicinal properties. In addition to eating fresh garlic, you can also crush a few pieces of cloves of garlic, add olive oil, and then pour into the salad. You can also buy garlic capsules. It is an excellent way to get the main ingredients of garlic into your body. Look for products that contain allicin. It is one of the significant parts of garlic.

Be careful

Generally, garlic is safe if taken regularly. The risk is small but can occur if you eat large amounts of garlic every day. Consuming more than four carnations a day can affect the body's platelets and prevent blood clots from forming. About two weeks before each SURGERY AND WHEN TAKING ANTICOAGULANTS, GARLIC CONSUMPTION SHOULD REDUCE.

GINGER

Ginger root

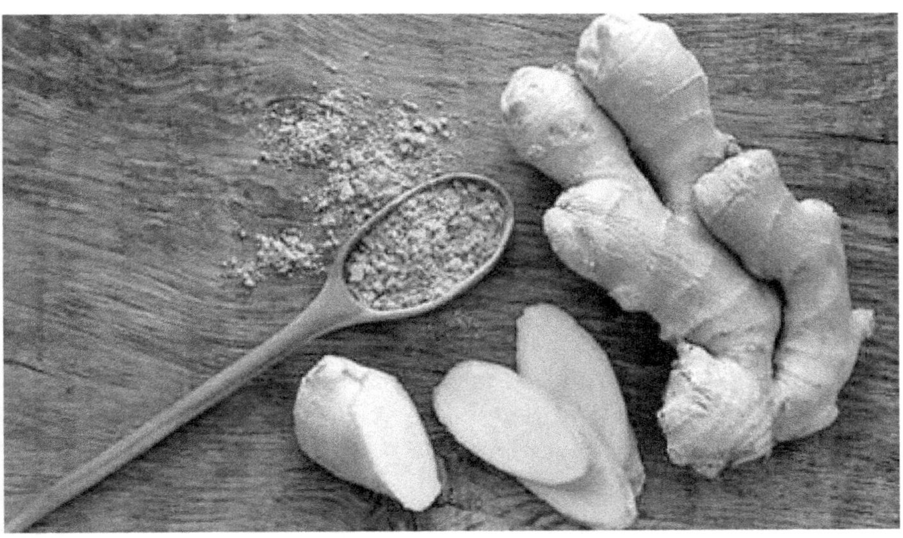

Ginger is a common herb used in cooking. It comes from Asia and has applied for over 4,400 years. In ancient times, it has used for Indian, Chinese, and Arabic medicine. It has so highly valued in the Middle Ages that he thought it came from the Garden of Eden. Today, ginger has used to treat problems related to motion sickness. Tea is also made from roots to cure many diseases. Greeks and Romans are the first to introduce ginger to Europe more than 2000 years ago. It was probably due to trade across the Arabian Peninsula.

Important medical applications

Motion sickness

inflammation

Cough and cold

Morning sickness

Nausea and vomiting

Antiemetic

Antioxidant

Circulation stimulant

Anti-inflammatory

Stimulates sweating

Peptic tonic

HOW TO USE:
Ginger root

Fresh ginger root

To treat a cold or cough, cut ginger root into 1-inch pieces, add 2 cups of water and simmer for 15 minutes to make a delicious ginger tea. Ginger, like many other herbs, is contained in capsules and is a great way to maintain ginger levels for the day. Extracts are also available but are generally only used to treat osteoarthritis.

Be careful

Ginger is a very safe herb but can cause heartburn. Besides, high doses of ginger and anticoagulants should not be combined.

GINKGO BILOBA

Ginkgo leaves

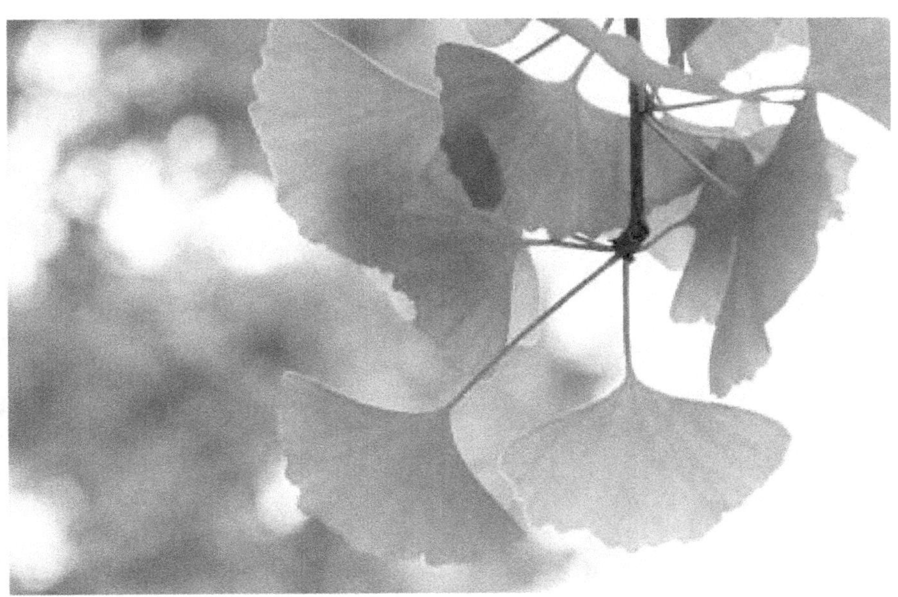

Ginkgo Biloba has used in Chinese medicine for thousands of years. Probably the first used by the Chinese, it is now widely used in both the United States and Europe. Ginkgo comes from ginkgo leaves but is perhaps not a herb to plant in the garden. I still think it's a beautiful herb that needs to add to our herbal list. Over the years, Ginkgo Biloba has built a reputation for beneficial to the brain. Two significant components of Ginkgo are flavonoids and terpenoids, both of which are antioxidants. Flavonoids have shown to help protect nerves, hearts, and blood vessels. Terpenoids are probably places where Ginkgo gains a reputation for being beneficial to the brain. Terpenoids enhance blood flow to the brain by expanding blood vessels and preventing platelets from sticking together.

Important medical applications

Mental health/performance

Antioxidant

Improve blood circulation

Protects nerve tissue

HOW TO USE:
Ginkgo capsule

Ginkgo capsule

As mentioned earlier, Ginkgo helps increase blood flow to the brain. Therefore, it is only natural that this herb can support cognitive function and memory. It has shown to help with symptoms related to the central nervous system, such as tinnitus and dizziness. The only place Ginkgo increases blood flow is not the brain. Consuming herbs from toes to the head increases blood flow throughout the body. Ginkgo is most often taken orally via a capsule. These are available at reasonable prices from Walgreens, CVS, and more.

Warning

Don't take Ginkgo if you are taking medication to prevent blood clotting. Also, stop using Ginkgo at least three days before surgery.

LAVENDER

Lavender field

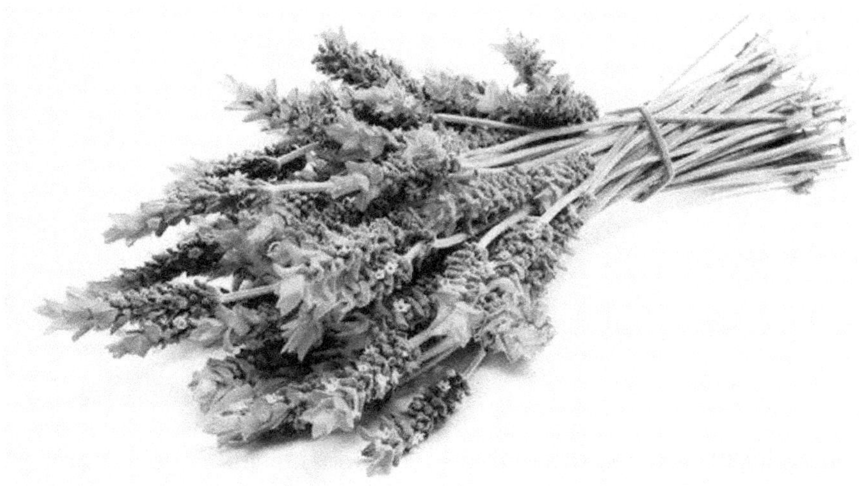

Lavender is probably best known for its aroma and is a beautiful herb for stressful days. Lavender is often used as a soap, detergent, or only as an essential oil, due to the soothing effect of the aroma. For the same reason, lavender is also widely used in tea. Lavender is quite old, dating back to the Mediterranean about 2500 years ago. Today, it is mainly grown for use as an essential oil. Lavender has many other applications for cooking as well as brewing tea with lavender. Lavender can add a slightly sweet floral taste. It works well with seafood, soups, salads, and baked goods.

Important medical applications

Antidepressant

Sedative effect

Preservative

Painkillers

Relieve gas

Antispasmodics

HOW TO USE:
Lavender essential oil

Lavender essential oil

As I said, lavender has often used in essential oils. The sedative, sedative, and relaxing effects of lavender oil make it ideal for headaches. You can add something to the handmade soap or put a few drops in the bathtub. I like using a humidifier and putting a few drops in a medicine bowl. That is a great way to raise lavender oil into the air and keep the room moist. Lavender oil applies to massage into the skin to relieve pain. Tea is also a great way to take advantage of lavender. When soaking tea, put a few cups of lavender twigs in a container and absorb quickly.

Be careful

Lavender is a very safe herb, but it has not recommended taking essential oils directly because it can cause unwanted side effects.

LEMON BALM

Lemon balm herb

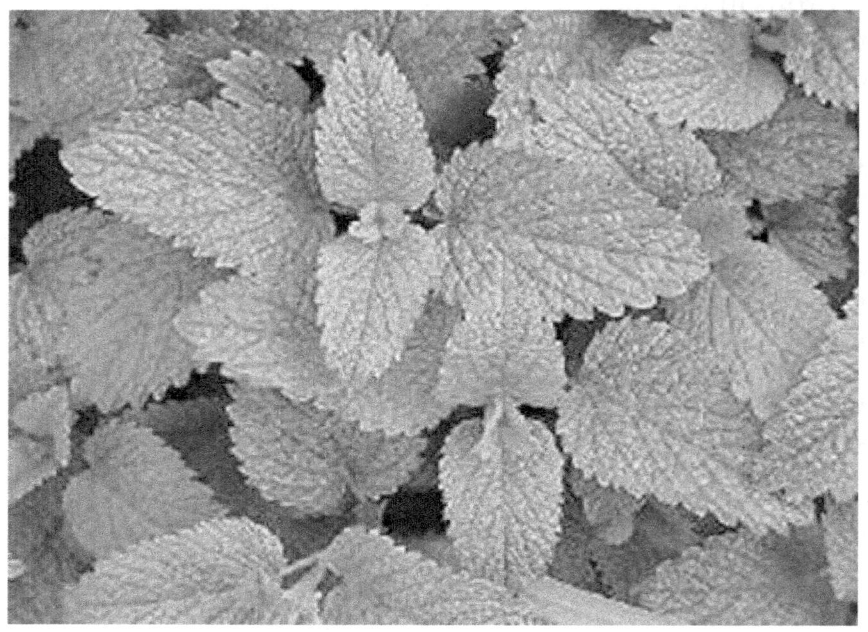

Lemon balm is a fragrant herb. By rubbing the leaves, it has a subtle mint and lemon-like aroma. Lemon balm was first used by the Greeks more than 2000 years ago and has long used in herbal medicine. At that time, both Greeks and Romans utilized lemon balm and wine to relieve the heat. Today, Lemon Balm works with other herbs, such as valerian and hops, to promote sleep and relax. Several studies have shown that it improves learning and memory. No wonder many herbal therapists recommend lemon balm to treat Alzheimer's disease.

Important medical applications

Bug spray

Antispasmodics

Relieve gas

Relaxing agent

Antiviral agent

Antidepressant

Fear and stress

Lemon balm tea

Lemon balm tea

There are several ways to apply the lemon balm. Lemon balm is a versatile herb, both in terms of the disease that has treated and how it administered. Tea is a great way to take advantage of lemon balm. Soak 5-6 fresh leaves in a glass of water for 6 minutes and strain. Add honey or stevia to sweeten the store, add a bit of mint and add more flavor. Tinctures, extracts, and ointments are also widely used in lemon balm and are all very useful.

NEEM

Neem goes

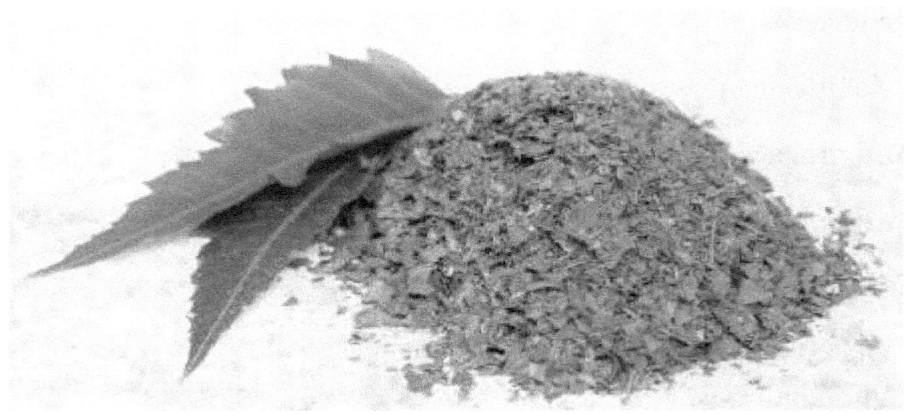

Neem has a long history as a medicinal herb. The story goes from Nimes to one of the oldest texts known to humanity. Neem's properties have mentioned in several ancient Sanskrit languages, and the Neem Sanskrit word (Nimba) means "healthy." Neem is a tree, so it may be difficult to classify it as an herb, but it couldn't remove from the herb list.

Given that everyone in India has been using Neem for over 4,000 years, there are things to consider when it comes to herbs. Today, neems have applied for several reasons, including skin treatments for eczema, scabies, head lice, and psoriasis. Neem is known not only for skin but also for hair.

Important medical applications

Blood purifier

Lowers blood sugar

antibacterial

Antifungal

Relieve itching

Anti-inflammatory

Support the immune system

How to use

Neem ointment in cans

Neem and vitamin E ointment

If using Neem as a skin toner, boil about 20 neem leaves in 0.5 liters of water. Once the leaves have become soft and discolored, and the water has turned green, the leaves have strained. Store the liquid in a bottle. If you want to use it, take a cotton ball, wet it with fluid, and put it on your face. It prevents acne and acne. Adding something to the bathwater can also prevent skin infections.

Be careful

You should give the children Neem locally. Lactating or pregnant women should not use Neem.

NETTLE

Nettle use

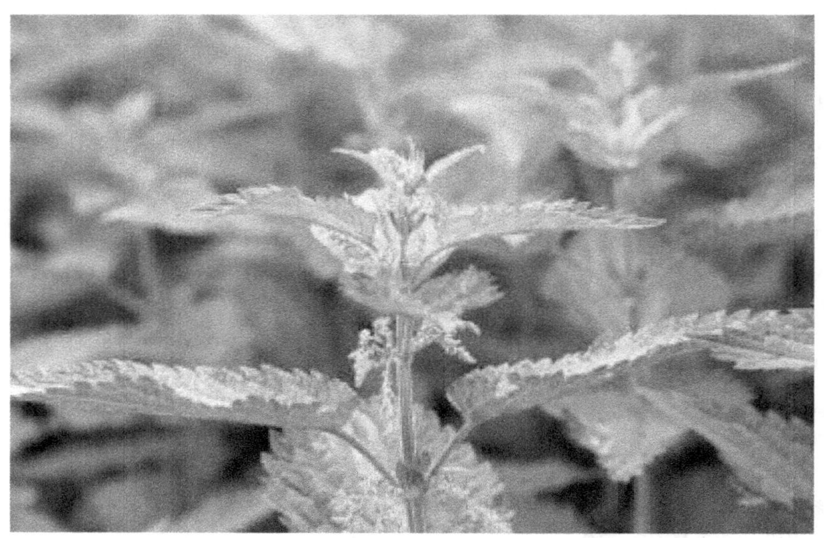

Nettle is a new herb common in Nebraska here. Nettle is probably best known you guessed it. Stinging nettle plants exhibit sharp spines upon contact and release a mixture of chemicals into the body once they penetrate the victim's skin. This is where the burning / itchy feeling occurs. Nettle plants release a combination of histamine, acetylcholine, serotonin, and formic acid. Surprisingly, the cure for this sting has found the plant itself. Juice from nettle leaves has applied to the affected area. Aside from the painful pain of nettle plants, it is a beneficial herb and deserves to be listed here.

Important medical applications

Antiallergic

Diuretic

Antispasmodics

Anti-inflammatory

Blood purifier

tonic

HOW TO USE:
Nettle leaf sack

1 pound bag of net leaves

Nettle plants have used in several ways. Tea, capsules, tinctures, and extracts are the best ways to utilize nettle. The tablet has used to treat hay fever symptoms. Generally, 300-800 mg has recommended. Tea has often consumed to achieve the strong diuretic effect of nettle. Due to this diuretic effect, it has used for arthritis, prostate health, high blood pressure, etc.

Be careful

Nettles have several side effects that you should be aware of. Upset stomach, rash, and impotence may occur but are rare. If anyone is taking medications for high blood pressure, diabetes, anxiety, or insomnia, consult your doctor before taking nettle herbs.

OREGANO

Oregano herb

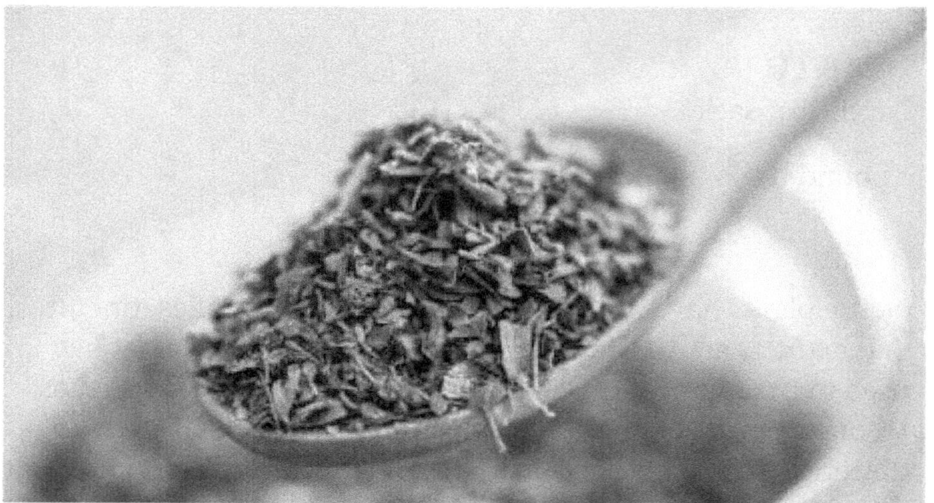

Another culinary herb creates a herbal list. Oregano is at the top of my list of culinary herbs. I love this. Oregano belongs to the Mint tribe, which has derived from the temperate climate of Eurasia and the Mediterranean. Oregano has first used by the ancient Greeks and believed that it has created by the goddess Aphrodite. Oregano comes from two Greek words. The first Oros means "Mountain," and the second Gano says "Joy," "Joy of the Mountain." It was until the Middle Ages that Oregano started as a herb and used herbs to treat toothache, rheumatism, indigestion, and cough.

Important medical applications

Antifungal

Expectorant

Stimulant

Preservative

Antioxidant

HOW TO USE:

Oregano oil

Undiluted oil

As you can imagine, Oregano has a long list of ways to use it in the kitchen. These are all great options, but besides adding to pasta dishes, you can do a lot with Oregano. Then make tea. This is an excellent way to lessen the time to recover from a disease. Oregano oil, diluted in coconut or olive oil, can be used topically to treat ringworm, athlete's foot, and warts.

Be careful

Oregano is high for many, but some people will find their skin irritated with oil. For this reason, test the water with a small amount of water and use only diluted oregano oil.

PEPPERMINT

Use peppermint herb

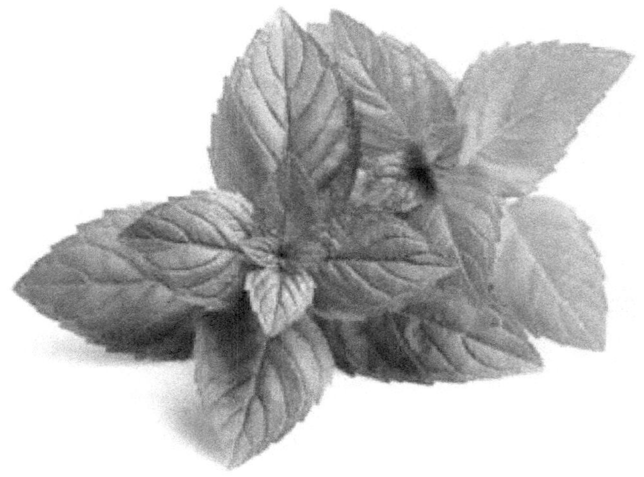

Peppermint is a very well-known herb today because of its fantastic scent when squeezed leaves. It has used in many different ways, both in cooking and medicinal, that it is hard to keep peppermint out of our herbal list. Peppermint originally came from England in the late 17th century and is a hybrid derived from water mint and spearmint. Peppermint was also widely used in ancient Egypt, which has applied for indigestion. Even dried peppermint leaves have found in pyramids built by Egyptians. In the 18th century, peppermint became popular in Western Europe for treating nausea, morning sickness, and respiratory infections.

Important medical applications

Relieve gas

Somewhat bitter

Mild sedative

Preservative

sweating

Mild painkillers

Antispasmodics

HOW TO USE:

Peppermint oil

Peppermint oil

Peppermint is the perfect herb to fight flu and colds. Peppermint can relieve sore throat symptoms by cooling and reducing sore throat. This is due to the menthol contained in Pfeffer.

PLANTAIN

Plantain

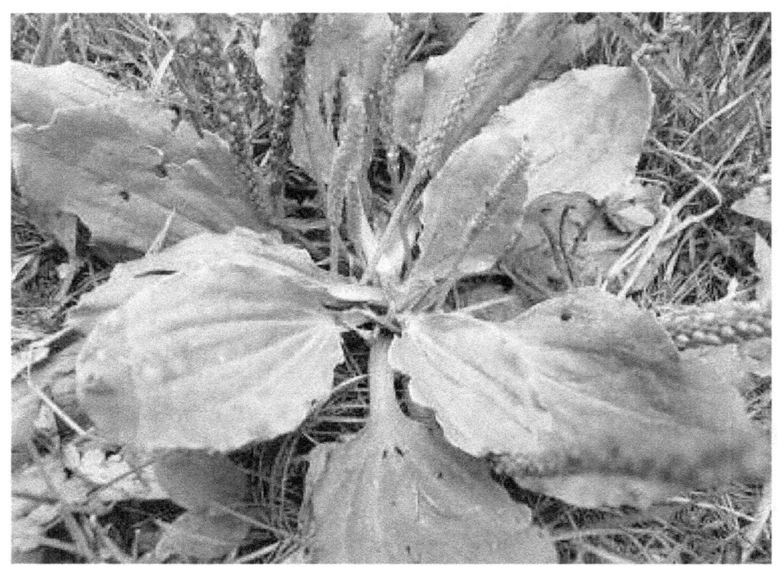

Plantain is probably one of the first herbs to reach the United States from Europe. Initially introduced by Puritan settlers, Wegerich was referred to by Native Americans as "the footprints of white men" because it could thrive were new settlers planted. Plantain grows around the world and is today considered a weed. However, it has some powerful medical benefits that should not overlook. In medieval Europe, the ability of psyllium to heal wounds such as cuts, burns, and swelling has already has established. It is not only a powerful wound healing psyllium but also shows promising results in the treatment of diseases such as edema, jaundice, ear infections, ringworm, and shingles. The significant components of psyllium leaf wax that contribute to the healing properties of psyllium are ocubin, melatonin, mucus, flavonoids, caffeic acid, and alcohol. All of this makes the essentials of your herb first aid kit.

Important medical applications

Wound healer

Painkillers

Antique catarrh

Anti-bleeding

Anti-inflammatory

Painkillers

Antiviral agent

How to use

Plantain leaf

4 oz pouch with plant leaves

Plantain has a relatively long list of uses that can treat acne by applying an ointment or tincture to the area. Shredding leaves can lead to effective sunburn treatment. These two uses alone prove that psyllium is an excellent herb for all preppers, but psyllium's benefits don't stop there. Plantains can heal cuts by healing cuts, so they can know when they are in the wild and put them in herb first aid kits. Psyllium, when brewed with tea, can also be used to treat colds, flu, and respiratory infections.

SAGE

Sage herb

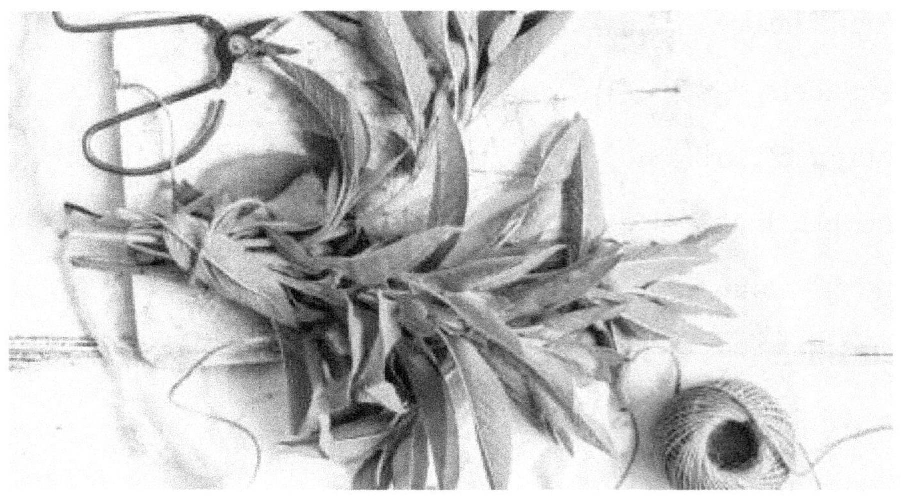

Sage also has some medicinal properties, like its most kitchen counterparts. It has features that help relieve sore throat, cough, and cold. Sage was used in ancient Egypt to prevent evil and snake bites and increase female fertility. In India, sage has used to manage sore throats and indigestion. Sage has been grown in gardens and kitchens since the Middle Ages, when the Romans introduced them to Europe. Today, sage has found in a variety of natural products that have sold. This makes sage an excellent herb for preppers, as these natural products can also have made. Deodorants have made from sage due to the properties of antiperspirants, and mouthwash is ordinary because sage can kill bacteria.

Important medical applications

Astringent

Antibacterial agent

Reduce sweating

estrogen

General tonic

Antioxidant

Peptic tonic

How to use

Organic sage tea

Organic sage tea

Tea is a great way to take advantage of sage. Just soak a teaspoon of sage in a glass of water for about 10 minutes. The combination of sage and thyme can also heal a sore throat. Put both in 1 oz and grind and cover with 16 oz apple cider vinegar. Shake regularly and rest for ten days before using it.

Be careful

A word of caution about sage, which contains a chemical called Quezon in its essential oils. Although safe for standard cooking applications, discretion has required at high doses, and alcohol extracts have not recommended.

SKULL CAP

Herbal skull cap

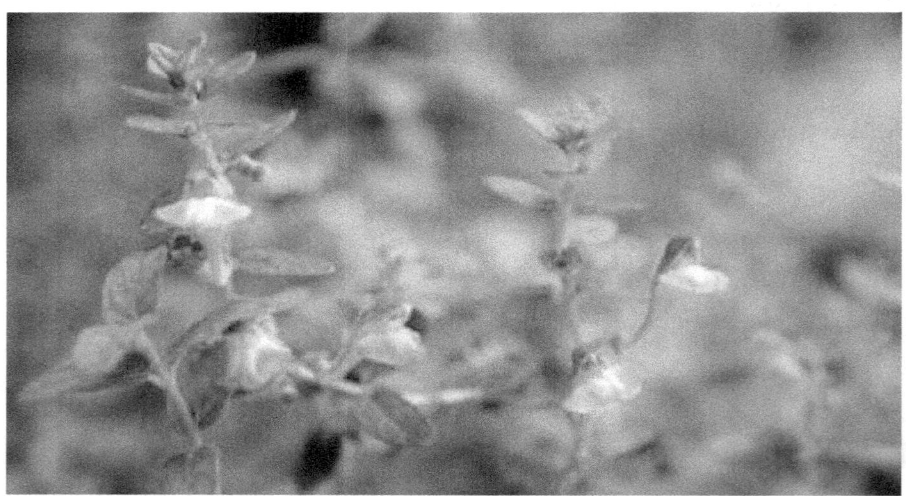

Skullcap is another herb of the mint family. The first medical use of skullcaps can probably have found by examining Native American life. The skull root has used as a treatment for diarrhea and kidney problems. Skullcaps became known as sedatives only when settlers arrived. They used it for every question, including fever, anxiety, and even rabies. Today, the upper part of the skull has most commonly used as a mild relaxing agent for anxiety, insomnia, tension headaches, and fibromyalgia. When it is growing skullcaps for herbal gardens, you need to be aware that there are both North American and Chinese varieties. Chinese skullcap is a much more difficult variety, grows well in both warm and cold climates, and withstands drought.

Important medical applications

Sedative

Somewhat bitter

Nervous tension

Antispasmodics

How to use

Skull cap capsule

Skull cap capsule

Skullcap tea has made by soaking a 1 oz skullcap in 50 liters of boiling water for about 10 minutes. Drinking this in a 1/2 cup dose every few hours will relieve headaches and anxiety. Also, if you don't have time to brew tea, this is a great way to use the skullcap right away.

Be careful

Use caution when using skull caps. It is a potent herb. Some reports suggest liver damage. Never use a skullcap if you have liver problems.

TURMERIC

Turmeric root

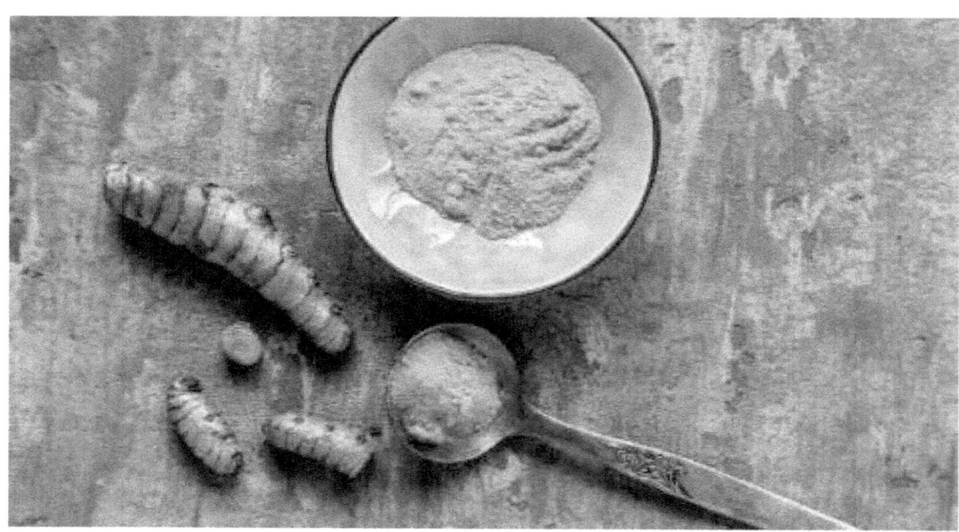

It tastes more like spices than herbs, but I had to add turmeric to the list of herbs. Turmeric has a long tradition in Hinduism and is related to purity and refining. Even today, Hindu brides attend a ceremony covering their faces with turmeric paste before vowing. Marco Polo once described turmeric as a vegetable with properties similar to saffron. It has only in the mid-twentieth century that Westerners recognized the benefits of turmeric. Curcumin is the main component of turmeric that provides these benefits. Turmeric has a curcumin concentration of about 3%. Therefore, it is more beneficial to take turmeric extract.

Important medical applications

Protects the liver

Antioxidant

Anti-inflammatory

How to use

Turmeric powder

1 LB bag turmeric

One of the best-known ways to use turmeric is to eat it. It may not be easy, but it's a great way to add it to your dishes. Don't be fooled by the fact that eating turmeric with food is the only way to take advantage of this beautiful herb. It has used as tea or toothpaste. Occasionally, brush your teeth with a toothbrush soaked in turmeric powder and rest for about 3 minutes. It does not stain your teeth, but the same does not apply to a toothbrush or sink. One can also make a turmeric paste by mixing turmeric powder with water and using it topically.

VALERIAN

Valerian herbs

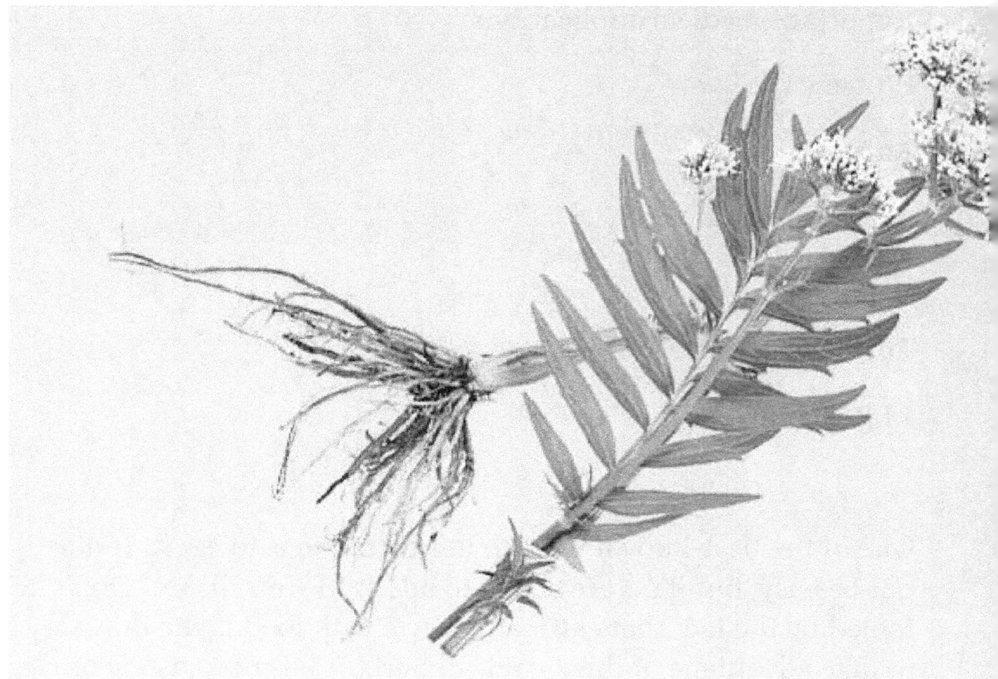

My personal favorite for promoting relaxation should be the
Valerian root. Valerian, like many others in this herbal list, was
first used by Greeks and Romans probably centuries ago. They
used Valerian to treat diseases of the liver, urinary tract, and
gastrointestinal tract. Valerian has once used to manage people
suffering from the plague. Your cat will love Valerian too! People
use Valerian just as we use catnip today. Some have said that the
effectiveness of Valerian has determined by the cat's response to
the herbs. Rats are not only cats that contain attractants but also
because of the stench that used to used in mousetraps. Today,

Valerian root is most commonly used as a sleep aid and dietary supplement to relieve anxiety.

Important medical applications

Mild painkillers

Somewhat bitter

Sedative

Antispasmodics

How to use

Valerian root capsule

Valerian root capsule

If anyone is looking for a better night's sleep, this is what I do: I take 2-3 valerian root capsules with 5 mg of melatonin, and it gives me a good night's sleep Does a perfect job. It's not overwhelming, but it helps me put myself in this sleep mode and stay there all night.

Be careful

Valerian has generally considered relatively safe, but there are some side effects to watch out for. Discontinue use if you have a headache, nausea, or pain in the upper stomach. Other less serious side effects include brain fog, dry mouth, strange dreams, and drowsiness.

WITCH HAZEL

Witch hazel

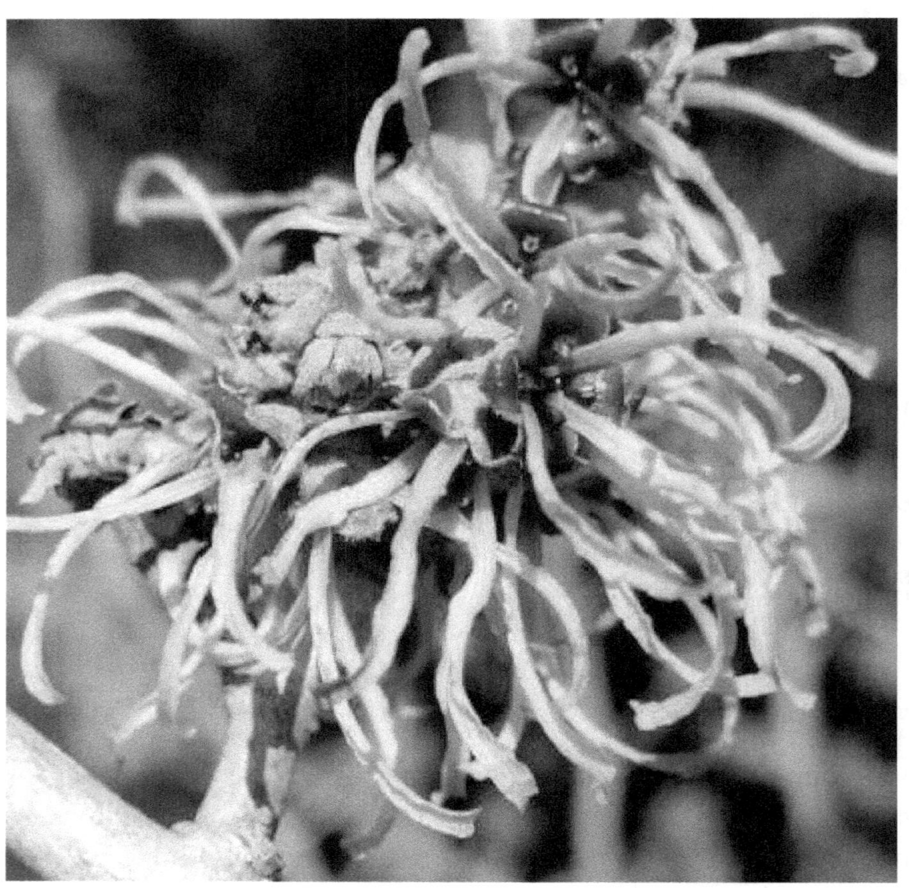

Witch hazel is a new herb that I just learned recently. However, it has been used by Native Americans for centuries. When studying Witch Hazel, I thought it had given its name, such as to repel the witch, but it was used as a witch's wand to find underground water sources and valuable minerals. Although witch hazel is a woody shrub, it may not be considered an herb by some, but it has a very strong astringency and antiseptic properties, so the list of herbs explains how to use it. I just added them. Today, almost all drugstores can find witch hazel in the form of witch hazel water (alcoholic extract of branches). The problem with this is, in most cases, the extracts contain very little of the herbs themselves, and most effects have attributed to the alcohol itself.

Important medical applications

Anti-inflammatory

Helps stop bleeding

Astringent

How to use

Witch hazel tonic

THAYER'S WITCH-HAZEL

Probably the easy way to use witch hazel is to make it tonic. You will need a witch hazel arc, distilled water, and half a pound of vodka: mix witch hazel and enough water to cover about 1-2 inches of bark. When boiling, cover and simmer for about 20 minutes. Next, sift the bark, add half of the tea to alcohol, and remove the bark. If you have 20 ounces of beverage, add 10 ounces of juice. Thayer toners are also suitable if you just want to make them in advance. Aloe vera has also included.

YARROW

Yarrow herb

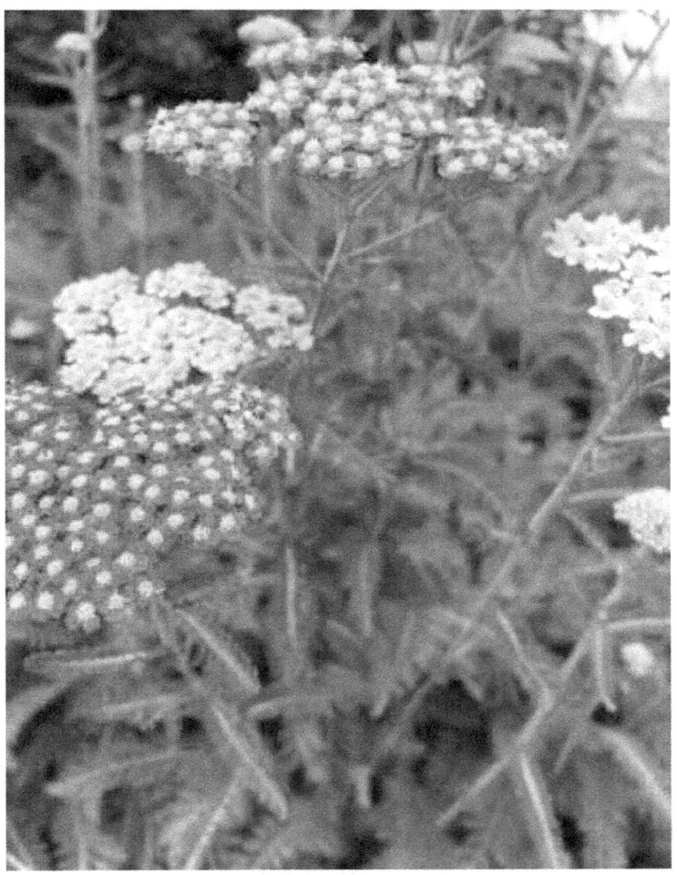

Yarrow is an excellent herb for herb, the first ID kit. It works to stop blood flow from a small cut. It has also used to cure bruises and relieve symptoms associated with colds, chimneys, and fever. Indians usedYarroww and called it "biomedical." They used it to treat earache and toothache as well. Achilles from Greece is said to have used Yarrow to heal soldiers during the Trojan War. Yarrow Achillea is actually derived from the name Achilles. Since many people in human history have used Yarrow as a spare herb, I decided to add it to our list of herbs.

Important medical applications

Astringent

Peptic tonic

Strengthens blood vessels

Stop bleeding

Wound healer

Stimulates sweating

Reduce fever

How to use

Yarrow tea

Sheep tea

A great way to take advantage of ofYarroww is to consume it as tea. This has used to reduce fever and reduce recovery time for colds and chimneys. Yarrows can also be made into creams or ointments and applied to small cuts that slow or stop bleeding.

Be careful

Do not use yarrows if you are pregnant or nursing. In rare cases, Yarrow has shown to cause allergic reactions, especially to the skin.

The number of patients seeking alternative or herbal remedies is growing exponentially. Herbal medicine combines the treatment experience of multiple generations of practitioners in the indigenous medical system for hundreds of years. In addition to being inexpensive, herbal medicines are highly receptive to culture, highly compatible with the human body. They have few side effects, so there is a strong demand for necessary medical care in developing countries today. However, recent evidence may indicate that not all herbal medicines are safe because of the severe effects reported for some herbal medicines. Most herbal products on the market today do not undergo a drug approval process to demonstrate safety and efficacy. Millennial traditional use can provide valuable guidelines for the selection, preparation, and use of herbal preparations. To be accepted as an alternative to modern medicine, the same rigorous scientific and clinical validation methods must use to demonstrate the safety and efficacy of therapeutic products. The current overview describes the present scenario and attempts to predict the future of Chinese herbal medicine.

Differences between traditional Chinese medicines and conventional medicines Although superficially similar, there are three critical differences between traditional Chinese drugs and traditional Chinese medicines: whole plant use-herbalists usually do not include several different ingredients. Use purified plant extracts. These have claimed to be able, act synergistically; the effect of the whole herb is more than the sum of the results of its ingredients. The use of whole herbs instead of isolated actives ("buffering") has also claimed to reduce toxicity. Two samples of a particular herbal medicine may contain ingredients in different proportions, but practitioners claim that this generally does not cause clinical problems. There is experimental evidence that certain herbal supplements have synergistic and buffering effects, but it is unclear to what extent this applies to all herbal products (Vickers and Zollman, 1999). Herbal Combinations-Several different herbs often used together. Practitioners argue that the principle of synergy and buffering applies to plant combinations and that herbal blends improve efficacy and reduce adverse effects. This is in comparison to traditional practices where polypharmacy has generally avoided where possible (Vickers and Zollman, 1999). Diagnostics-Herbal practitioners use different diagnostic principles than conventional practitioners. For example, when treating arthritis, you can observe that the patient's excretory symptoms are not working correctly and determine that the arthritis is due to the "accumulation of metabolic waste." Second, a combination of herbal diuretics, bile, or laxatives, in addition to herbs containing antidiabetic drugs, can prescribe inflammatory properties (Vickers and Zollman, 1999). The evidence of human use of plants for healing why people use herbal medicine dates back to the Neanderthal era (Winslow and Kroll, 1998). Currently, an increasing number of patients do not usually report concurrent use of herbal medicines to clinicians (Miller, 1998). There are several reasons patients turn to herbal remedies. Often referred to as "control, mental comfort from behavior" that explains why many people who take herbs have a chronic or incurable illness. Diabetes, Cancer, Arthritis, or AIDS. In such situations, they often believe that conventional medicine has failed.

Herbal Drug Safety Issues Traditional herbal products are inherently heterogeneous. They pose several challenges for qualifying control, quality assurance, and regulatory processes. Most herbal products on the market today do not undergo a drug approval process to demonstrate safety and efficacy. Some of them contain mercury, lead, arsenic (Kew et al., 1993), and corticosteroids (De Smet, 1997) and harmful amounts of toxic organic substances. Liver failure and even death after taking Chinese herbs have reported (Chattopadhyay, 1996). Prospective studies have shown that 25% of corneal ulcers in Tanzania and 26% of blindness in children in Nigeria and Malawi are associated with the use of traditional ophthalmic drugs (Harries and Cullinan, 1994). The side effects of some medicinal plants are under investigation (Gupta and Raina, 1998). Sometimes patients use traditional and traditional medicines at the same time. The in vivo interaction of these two drugs can be dangerous and can raise serious concerns about patient safety among physicians (Chattopadhyay, 1997). If the patient is taking conventional medicine, herbal preparation should be used with extreme care and only with the advice of a herbal expert familiar with the relevant traditional pharmacology. There have been cases of serious adverse events following the administration of herbal products.

In most cases, the herbs involved has prescribed and purchased over-the-counter or obtained from sources other than registered practitioners. Recently, several women developed rapidly progressing interstitial renal fibrosis after consuming a herbal medicine prescribed at a slimming clinic (Vickers and Zollman, 1999). Belgian physicians have recently discovered that the Chinese herb Aristolochia fang chi is not only associated with renal failure but can also cause cancer (Kew et al., 1993). After dozens of diet physicians at the weight loss clinic developed symptoms of renal failure, the study found that Belgian pharmacists were misusing them labeled Chinese herbal medicine to assemble a diet drug (Greensfelder, 2000). As more people use herbal medicine, pharmacists must be informed about their safety. This requires an assessment of the market coverage and regulations of products that may affect product safety (Boullata and Nace, 2000). The adverse effects of some traditional Chinese medicines have recently has investigated (Yi-Tsan and Chuang-Ye, 1997).

Most of the Ayurvedic preparations available on the market are wrong, tampered with, or have the wrong brand (Kumar 1998). Most of the developments on the market do not even support old Ayurvedic texts. One year after giving birth, it is medicinal, powders made from them are only valid for six months, and pastes are valid for one year. However, formulations usually do not have an expiration date or potential side effects.

In some cases, you can see that almost all herbal medicines mixed with symptomatic drugs. LeicesterRoyalInfimary found that a sample of traditional Chinese medicine given to women for eczema contained steroids (Graham-Brown et al., 1994).

Undeclared medications, including phenylbutazone, diazepam, and corticosteroids, have been demonstrated in traditional Chinese arthritis treatments (Vander Stricht et al., 1994).

Without control, there is no guarantee that herbs contained in the bottle will be the same as those listed on the outside. The widespread neglect of quality control in the health food industry has undermined the production of many essential herbs. For example, it has estimated that over 50% of Echinacea sold in the United States between 1980 and 1991 was parthenium integrifolium due to the detection of a supplier error.

This emphasizes the importance of using the scientific name Latin because both herbs above are called "Snakeroot, Missouri" and have applied for proper plant identification based on sensory, microscopic, and technical analysis (Murray and Pizzahorno, 2000). Plant materials used in industrial and developing countries as raw materials for home remedies, over-the-counter medicines, and the pharmaceutical industry.